overcoming
distractions

overcoming distractions

Thriving with Adult
ADD/ADHD

DAVID A. GREENWOOD

STERLING
New York

STERLING
New York

An Imprint of Sterling Publishing Co., Inc.
1166 Avenue of the Americas
New York, NY 10036

ISBN 978-1-4549-2076-2

Library of Congress Cataloging-in-Publication Data

Names: Greenwood, David A., author.
Title: Overcoming distractions / David A. Greenwood.
Description: New York : Sterling, 2016.
Identifiers: LCCN 2016020744 | ISBN 9781454920762
Subjects: LCSH: Attention-deficit disordered adults. | Attention-deficit
  hyperactivity disorder. | Distraction (Psychology) | Time management.
Classification: LCC RC394.A85 G745 2016 | DDC 616.85/89--dc23
LC record available at https://lccn.loc.gov/2016020744

Distributed in Canada by Sterling Publishing Co., Inc.
ᶜ/o Canadian Manda Group, 664 Annette Street
Toronto, Ontario, Canada M6S 2C8
Distributed in the United Kingdom by GMC Distribution Services
Castle Place, 166 High Street, Lewes, East Sussex, England BN7 1XU
Distributed in Australia by NewSouth Books
45 Beach Street, Coogee, NSW 2034, Australia

For information about custom editions, special sales, and
premium and corporate purchases, please contact Sterling Special Sales
at 800-805-5489 or specialsales@sterlingpublishing.com.

Manufactured in Canada

2 4 6 8 10 9 7 5 3 1

www.sterlingpublishing.com

Author photo: Matt Baldelli Photograph

DEDICATED TO MY WIFE EMILY
who has always allowed me to chart my own
course in life

AND MY SON NATHANIEL
who will someday show the world that being
different can be a gift.

CONTENTS

Why does a book like this need to be written?

I'll give you several reasons. First, take a few minutes and Google the phrase "What is ADHD?" Here's the answer: It's Attention Deficit Hyperactivity Disorder. But as you scroll down, you'll find one of the first reasons this book needs to be written: Many of the initial search results speak about children. They describe ADHD as a childhood disorder or childhood illness. The word "illness" gets to me, but more on that later. Even the National Institute of Mental Health calls ADHD a childhood disorder and barely mentions the word "adult."

Pages and pages of many credible websites speak to the condition as being a childhood issue and not so much something that adults experience. It may be much more noticeable in children than in adults. And I get why many of these entries, articles, websites, books, and other publications focus on childhood ADHD. It's difficult to watch your child struggle with behavior, schoolwork, getting along with others, and all the casualties that go along with being a kid with ADHD, including bullying.

It's estimated that 10 percent of school-aged children show some of the most recognized traits of ADHD, including focus and behavioral issues, hyperactivity, and impulsivity. Or, as I like to say, they have "no filter."

Raising a child with ADHD is not easy. It's stressful, exhausting, and turbulent all at the same time. I know because I'm raising a child with his own challenges. My wife likes to say that my mother is looking down on me from heaven now and giving me just a little bit of a payback for everything I put her through when I was a kid.

Some days I do feel that I'm reliving my childhood, and not always in a good way.

Now I'm an adult, running a small business and raising a child with extreme focus issues. You'd probably love to be a fly on the wall in our house.

Over the years I've had my good days and bad days, but overall I was always, as an adult, driven to succeed. As a teenager I probably could not have cared less about being successful. I was only concerned about hanging out at the corner store with friends and driving my red Trans Am down to the beach. But something finally clicked in my early twenties, and I was suddenly determined to be successful in some way, making up for the complete disaster that was my formal education. I didn't go to crappy schools—I was just a crappy student.

Guess what? Kids with ADHD grow up to be adults with ADHD. Stunning, I know. Maybe we learn to deal with it, but how do we *thrive* with ADHD? That was my question when I finally decided to get my act together.

As adults, many of us can either mask the symptoms of ADHD or, as we get older, hide them in certain situations. But the fact remains that many kids who have ADHD grow up with it and struggle with it on a daily basis. And many decide to kick a little ass with it and become successful adults.

One of those kids is me. Although, when I was growing up, it wasn't called ADHD. Kids like me were classified as simply "hyperactive." In my case, hyperactive would be more than an accurate description. And the schools had absolutely no idea what to do with us. As you'll read in these pages, some of the people I interviewed for this book were even thrown out of school. In my case, I'm quite confident that I inadvertently tortured my mother, my teachers, and others with my behavior. And I'm not quite sure my grandparents understood me at all.

But I think I made up for it. Before my mother passed away, I owned and grew two successful businesses and took on a high-profile role at a well-known charity, often acting as a spokesperson for national and international events.

I knew that there were people out there just like me, and even those with symptoms like mine who far exceeded my success. And I wanted to get to know them. I wanted to tell their stories, and I wanted to show the world that the kid in your classroom you thought was a complete screwup now runs a very successful business and might even be making much more money than you are. He may have also invented something that changed an industry, the world, and even your life. As one person puts it in this book, it may be juvenile, but many of us have something to prove.

But the deeper issue is this: How can we learn from these successful people? What drives them? What gets them out of bed in the morning, and what keeps them motivated to go for it every day? I wanted to know, and so do many of my fellow ADHDers who are looking for ways not only to make it through the day, but also to rise above their ADHD and make it work in their favor. We have to fight to figure out what to do with ourselves after our feet hit the floor in the morning, getting our brains and body into a zone that gets us through the day.

In writing this book, I talked to many people, including successful business owners, those who are successful in their respective careers, as well as ADHD coaches and a handful of highly regarded medical professionals in the field of ADHD. *Overcoming Distractions* is meant to be a street-smart approach to managing and thriving with ADHD. It's not meant to be a medical book or to offer doctors' advice. Since I went to a vocational school for welding, I'm far from a medical doctor. And while ADHD is formally classified as a medical condition of the brain, I don't believe the answers to living a great life lie solely in medical solutions.

Successful people learn how to manage their environment and adapt, and that is no different than what someone with ADHD does to succeed. We can't go to school and learn how to be a successful businessperson with ADHD. We need to learn from screwing up, and from those who have done it, and we need to create techniques that allow us to thrive. And that's what this book offers.

If you're reading this book, you most likely have ADHD. And maybe sticking with things for the long haul, such as reading a book, isn't your thing. I get it. But stick with it. You'll meet some great people in this book and get some incredible advice that can help you crank up your career, your business, and turn what many people think of as a negative into an incredible positive in your life. I feel honored to have been given the opportunity to introduce you to the people whose stories you are about to hear and whose lessons you will learn from.

Most people in this book actually credit their ADHD with their success and are glad they have it. That might not have been the case growing up, but looking back, their creativity and innovation have been a result of their ADHD. And that's allowed them to become who they are today.

If you don't have ADHD and you just decided this might be a good book, I hope you find some of the advice of those with ADHD valuable enough to incorporate in your daily life. The list of those who have become super-successful and just happen to have ADHD continues to grow. From airline executives to professional athletes, political consultants, and many others, we can learn from those who have become super-successful. They must be doing something right.

One more thing before we start our journey. You will not find many references to medication here. While I do realize that medication is a part of managing your ADHD if you choose that route, I didn't want this to be a medical book. That being said, I do believe it's worth having an open and honest discussion with a doctor about whether you should be taking medication. And to bring that one step further, I believe you should consult a doctor who specializes in ADHD. Have your general practitioner refer you to an ADHD specialist. Medication, like anything else you learn about here, is your choice, to be discussed with your doctor. You don't have to if you don't want to, but it might help you. Some of those I spoke to swear by their medication and have difficulty functioning without it. Others have had a very bad experience with medication. I do not take any medication, and I am fine with that decision in my life. Might I find it easier to function with some type of ADHD medication? I may never know, but that's my choice.

Your choice to take ADHD medication is between you, your doctor, and your family.

But keep this in mind: Medication is not the sole answer to thriving with ADHD. Thriving with ADHD is the result of a collection of techniques, tools, and self-regulation that helps adults with ADHD become successful and dependable to others. And I hope you learn those tools from reading on.

Let's do this!

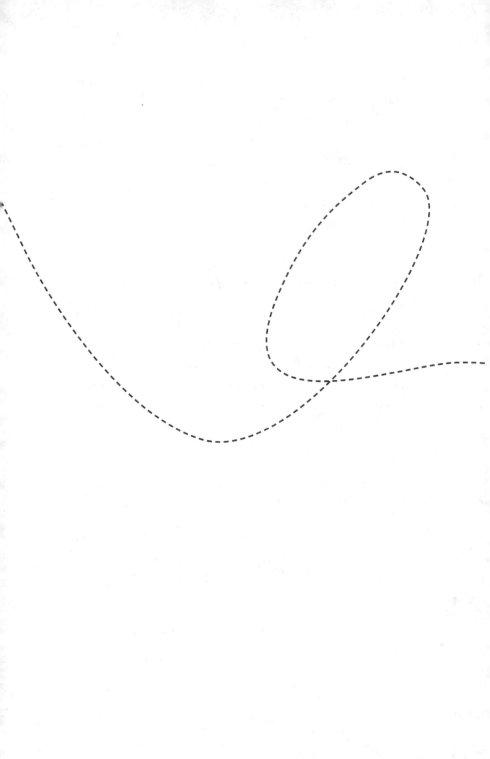

overcoming distractions

you will finish
this book . . .

So, have you ever purchased a book and then never picked it up? I know—you get all excited when you buy it or it comes in the mail. Maybe you read some of it or maybe not. Do you have a pile of books you never read? I'll make a confession right now: I'm one of those people. I have books that my family has given me for my birthday or Christmas, and they are still collecting dust.

So, what makes me think someone with ADHD is going to actually read a book about adult ADHD and how to thrive with it? Because it's written by one of your own—an adult with ADHD. And more importantly, the stories in this book are about people just like us. They know how to kick the hell out of ADHD as an adult and how to be a success in their business and career.

So I'll answer some questions right up front: Why did I write this book? And why should you read the entire book?

The short answer for those with ADHD who are thinking of putting this book down is that I wanted to know how others like you and me got to where they did, having the same type of brain I did. I wanted to know how they said, "Screw you, ADHD. I'm building a successful business." Oh, and to all those kids who made fun of me in school because I was different? Let's compare paychecks.

I wanted to know how people like me cut through the fog of ADHD and got stuff done! And, how did they get stuff done without totally relying on medication to manage their ADHD? What drives them, what motivates them, what helps them make every day count? And how do they handle a bad day? Because everyone has a bad day. Now, some people interviewed for this book do take medication, so again, I will not go down the road of saying all medication is bad. Both those I interviewed as well as coaches and doctors say that if you need medication, take it. But this book will outline how to use it in collaboration with other methods of managing your ADHD.

I wanted to somehow inspire others. For years I have hidden the fact that I never finished college. At parties, when others talked about their college days, I would stand there, smiling and nodding, playing along and letting people believe that I had had the same experiences as my friends. I joked about being ADHD, but never really made it more than a passing joke.

But then there were the people who were impressed by my accomplishments, never knowing that I crashed and burned at college. And even flunked out of freshman year at a vocational school. Who the hell flunks out of vocational school? Me, that's who. Can a vocational school dropout inspire others? I hope so!

I began to write this book after running my own PR and video marketing firm for several years. When I first started in the field of public relations, PR professionals were primarily responsible for getting media coverage. Yes, we did other things, such as write newsletters, produce an occasional video, and provide other collateral materials, but that's pretty much it. There were few other outlets for getting the word out. If we wanted to share a video of a cat hanging from a ceiling fan, we sent it to all our friends through email, faxed press releases to the media, and waited. Sounds like the Stone Age to us now, but that's how we made things go viral, if you will.

I was always a creative person, and having ADHD, PR was a great fit for my type of brain. I thought differently and was rewarded with great results in my chosen profession. I built a very successful restaurant business by being creative with PR, and after that, I managed the public relations for a very well-known charity and had even better results. I had found my calling. I loved what I did and got a thrill every time I saw a TV camera. For this ADHD guy who never finished college, I had finally found what I was good at. And, I might say, I was better at it than many.

Ideas would pop into my head, and in no time, I was planning the next way to get media coverage for the organization. Call it a knee-jerk reaction to inspiration or whatever you want, but for me, this dynamic worked, and ADHD was my friend. I really believe that if you harness the power of ADHD, it is a blessing. Yes, for many people, ADHD gets in the way of trying to achieve something, but if you embrace it, understand that there will be good days and bad, there is nothing you can't accomplish. And with the right support system, you can live a great life.

After starting my PR firm, social media began to take shape. Many of us were already using sites like LinkedIn, but none of us called them "social media." Facebook came along, and then Twitter, and public relations as we knew it slowly began to change. Through online public relations and our need to understand features like search engine optimization to get a client on the first page of Google results, an entire industry was changing. Talk about ADHD!

Many of us in the PR industry tried hard to keep up with the times. In the beginning, I had very good luck getting clients media coverage. But my old methods slowly started to become ineffective.

It's not that I was bad at the new dynamics of PR using social media. When I worked for Special Olympics, I saw more TV cameras in my career than most in my industry see in an entire lifetime, so I was well-versed in thinking on my feet, and I had a Rolodex of reporters and journalists that any PR person would die for. But the media landscape was changing, and getting clients traditional press coverage was getting harder.

Newspapers were getting thinner because of all the opportunities the Internet gave marketers. Entire media outlets were going out of business, and many media companies were laying off reporters by the dozens—reporters we in the PR business had spent so much time cultivating relationships with. The editor of my hometown newspaper once told me that she now was expected to edit two newspapers, two websites, lay off half her staff, and take a 25 percent pay cut just to keep afloat.

To save my business, I started to offer video production. I was using a great video company, but because of how things were changing, I realized that if I didn't change my business model, I would be out of business in the coming years.

I was no stranger to video, having produced several videos for Special Olympics and other clients, but I did have to teach myself how to shoot good video and edit. I did just that and, in the next few years, was making videos for almost all my clients. It got to the point where companies were hiring us just to do video marketing, something I really enjoyed. I ultimately started doing all our marketing around our video marketing services, getting away from traditional PR.

So now this ADHD guy was getting clients media coverage, managing social media such as Twitter and Facebook accounts, shooting and editing video, helping clients rank higher in search engine results, publishing email newsletters, and so on. My business was testing the bounds of my ADHD. How do other successful people in business manage their ADHD? I was asking this question constantly.

We were a very small PR firm, which meant I was managing the accounts of each and every client. I had writers and a full-time public relations specialist who did quite a bit for clients, but I had to oversee it all. As I'll outline in this book, multitasking does not work for most people—and, in my opinion, it's deadly for someone with ADHD. Then again, some people interviewed in this book say otherwise, that multitasking does work for them, and that they thrive on working on many tasks at once. But it wasn't a very good strategy for me.

As I was writing this book, Google and other search engines have made all kinds of changes to their systems that made many of our online PR tactics ineffective. Plus, every week another new social media platform seems to emerge, and even existing social media sites have changed the rules, so we have to constantly keep up with changes in the industry. It's enough to make your head spin. You tell a client we need to implement one kind of strategy and three months later—nope, we can't do that anymore. You get pissed and the client gets pissed. Plus, when you're doing it all with little help, it starts to make you a little overwhelmed.

So you can see so far that I'm juggling more and more balls in the air every day. All the changes in the PR and marketing industry were enough to test anyone with ADHD, including me. But I'm not done.

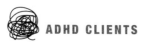 **ADHD CLIENTS**

First of all, I had the great fortune of having some tremendous clients. Many have stayed with me for years because of the quality of work we do. They have gone through the myriad changes in the public relations world, listened to my counsel, and rolled with the punches. I have always had a great working relationship with our clients, and if I think it's a bad fit, we part ways. It's too stressful to work with clients who are not a good fit.

While I have had wonderful clients, I have also had my share of clients where the entire organization operated like an ADHD kid. Those are the companies that can't speak with one voice. There are individuals who have symptoms of ADHD, and then there are entire organizations that are scatterbrained. Having my share of these clients was certainly stressful. One person asks you to do one project, you do it, and then another person asks why it was done. Or the company designates a person to sign off on projects, and his boss doesn't like the choice your liaison made. Better yet, your corporate contact asks where you are on a project, but she hasn't given you what you asked for months before. OK, maybe that's just corporate America. Anyway, it was making this ADHD guy feel his symptoms even more acutely.

The most common joke about those with ADHD is "Oh, look, a squirrel . . ." The implication is that people with ADHD are distracted by anything and can even be taken off course midsentence by the sight of an animal or other distractions. But here's what I would say to that: Sometimes that squirrel is a great idea running by us, and if we don't pay attention to it, we could lose sight of something that could make a tremendous difference in our business.

In this book I speak with many very successful people, some of whom you may know. I get inside their thought processes; I go back through their childhood; I find out how they manage their ADHD; and I learn how they grow their businesses. I also share some very funny stories about their life with ADHD. I share a few of mine as well, including just how hyper I was as a child and how I drove my mother nuts. Sound familiar?

Yes, those with ADHD will enjoy this book, but those without ADHD, those who are looking for the great stories behind successful people should discover life lessons as well. You'll meet people who might just have a few things in their way and think a little differently, but become and stay successful.

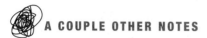

A COUPLE OTHER NOTES

Everyone has her own opinion. And you know what they say about opinions. We are all individuals, and what works for you, might not work for me. Some in this book—maybe even you—might need medication, while others are dead set against using any form of medication. Some may use vigorous exercise and meditation in place of drugs, and that works for them. Others use a combination of strategies to manage ADHD, which may or may not include medication. One person interviewed for this book had a horrific time getting off medication, while others use it just when they need to focus intently on a project. Just keep an open mind. This is by far not the bible on ADHD and all that claims to cure it. It's a collection of stories and advice to help and inspire you to take action in your own life.

Also, I use a couple different terms in this book. Many call what we are talking about now ADHD. But there are a few who refer to it as ADD. To quickly refresh your memory, ADD stands for Attention Deficit Disorder while ADHD stands for Attention Deficit Hyperactivity Disorder. The term and diagnosis have evolved over the years and are now more commonly referred to as ADHD. You will see throughout this book that I refer to it as ADHD, but if the person I have interviewed referred to it as ADD, I would hesitate to put words into his mouth. ADHD expert and best-selling author Dr. Edward Hallowell, whom you'll meet soon, doesn't like either term—"ADD" or "ADHD"—because he feels there are so many gifts that come with being who we are. There are positives and negatives to being ADHD, and the term only focuses on the negative.

While it may be slightly confusing, it's far better than what they called me and many others: "hyperactive children." Maybe we climbed the walls, stared out the window, and occasionally flipped over a desk in school, but we also had great abilities to dream big and see things that others could not envision. From what I remember of my childhood, they didn't really know what to do with kids like us. And then we grew up.

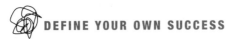 **DEFINE YOUR OWN SUCCESS**

While there are many success stories about those with ADHD, such as those who have built a business or several businesses, many people have defined their own success personally. If you are happy doing a job you love, and it nourishes your inner needs, then I would argue that you are successful. Just finding a career that you can do well in and contribute to a larger mission constitutes success for some of us. I spoke to many entrepreneurs and wildly creative people during this process, and I met several people who just love what they do and are not millionaires. They have overcome obstacles and work in careers they thought they might not be able to do. As I was writing this book, I received several emails with this message: "I don't know if I'm very successful." Well, you are successful if you have found a way to be happy and fulfilled in life.

Casey Dickson is one of those people I chatted with, and she's got a job that she's very proud of. She has ADHD as well as executive function disorder, which we will discuss in an upcoming chapter. She works at a nonprofit organization that assists individuals with disabilities who wish to gain work experience and ultimately work toward meaningful employment. Casey is the administrative office assistant and helps much of the organization stay organized, in addition to her other responsibilities. "I didn't even think of applying for administrative jobs," says Casey. She was looking more at retail jobs because that was the work experience she had. She also felt that she didn't have enough office or corporate experience on her resume to stand out among other applicants for administrative jobs. She had the required skills because she had helped out at her father's office, but didn't think she could compete with other candidates.

Casey handles the organization's social media, helps with payroll, answers phones, takes minutes for various conference calls, transcribes handwritten notes for coworkers, and is in charge of ordering supplies. She needs to be organized. For someone who might have challenges with time management, completing tasks, or keeping track of how long it takes to complete a task, Casey is doing an outstanding job. And she really likes her position and the fact that she's been given these responsibilities. She even receives regular commendations for her work from her boss. "I feel happy in the job; I feel like I'm accomplishing something; and I feel like my opinion is validated and valued."

I spent some time speaking with a woman named Pamela Curtis. She says she was never flagged as someone with ADHD when she was young because in most cases it was the boys who showed hyperactive behavior. "I was the kid who was always staring out the window, thinking of something entirely else than what was going on," says Pamela. But she feels that she did get a reputation in school for being "that kid." I think we all remember "that kid": the one who stood out in our classroom by actually not standing out.

Pamela was diagnosed with ADHD at the age of twenty-two, after getting out of college. She did learn coping skills from her father while in high school, but she was not officially diagnosed until some time had passed and she was still having trouble completing basic tasks and focusing. While her father helped her stay on target when doing schoolwork and helped her organize her life in other ways, when she set off on her own,

Pamela was having difficulty managing her life. She sought out professional help, at which point she received her diagnosis. One of the hardest things to do for those with ADHD is to just get started on a task or project, and her father had helped her with those time management skills.

Pamela gravitated toward writing and English while in college and was getting great grades in those classes. She ended up earning a degree in English and started a successful writing career. She had a love of computers and technology, and while working at a technology company, a coworker suggested she try her hand at technical writing. "My ADD became a strength rather than a weakness," says Pamela. And she leveraged that ADHD into technical writing. She ended up writing "how to" guides for various software programs and manuals on how hardware worked. As she puts it, "I translated geek-speaking into layman."

She is also the author of the book *Chin Up! 50 Ways to Make Money While Disabled*, in which she details how those with disabilities can earn income while dealing with a disability. She outlines several ways a person can earn a healthy living working from home—another accomplishment based on her writing skills.

Pamela developed a disability several years ago. She was experiencing constant migraine headaches, and it was determined that a rare pituitary disorder was affecting her thyroid and adrenal glands, causing the migraines. She has now transitioned to a career working as a disability advocate for a law firm, again using her writing and translation skills to her benefit and the benefit of others. Her new job is another great fit for her skills as a writer.

One way she stays productive is by recognizing that if the work appeals to her intellect and thrills her, she knows that she can be productive. She also says that it's important to give herself the freedom to be a person with ADHD and not look at it as a problem, but almost as a superpower. She feels that this type of thinking has been the biggest benefit to her. In her view, if you can be all over the place, as many ADHD people are, but still find a way to come back to the task at hand, you'll be successful.

One of the ways to do this is to find what you love. More often than not, a person with ADHD will be successful when he is interested in a job, career, or a business. And that also goes for individual tasks. For example, I hate doing bookkeeping, so I leave it to the last minute. But I love working closely with my clients, so that would take priority over my bookkeeping. I loved working on the PR and marketing for the restaurant I used to own, but I hated making hundreds of sandwiches every day.

Katharine Ligon is a mental health policy analyst in Austin, Texas, who loves what she does. She was diagnosed with ADHD at age seventeen, and school was very challenging to her. She barely remembers learning in school that wasn't, in some ways, painful. Katharine used humor to get through some of the lessons that she had a hard time with, but she also did well in the courses in which she had an interest. All in all, Katharine felt she needed to learn in a different way to be successful in school, and that was sometimes at odds with the way her classes were taught. At one parent-teacher conference in fifth grade, her teacher referred to her as "stupid," and her parents removed her from the school.

Her parents got her into a private school that provided education for children with learning disabilities. She was able to acquire new learning skills, as well as gain a grasp of reading comprehension. And in ninth grade, she went back to public school with some new skills. But Katharine soon learned that she needed additional support in order to graduate.

After reading the groundbreaking book *Driven to Distraction* by Dr. Edward Hallowell, as many in this book have done, she began to figure things out. She started taking Ritalin, which helped. She headed off to college, and after two years, decided to take some time off. She felt that she was not doing very well. She was working tremendously hard for mediocre grades, and it was just not satisfying to her.

She started doing youth ministry work and volunteering in Honduras for a home that worked with abandoned and abused girls. She was teaching classes and assisting the girls with their day-to-day living activities. "That really gave me a lot of purpose in life, gave me a lot of direction, and it gave me a perspective that I didn't have before."

After two years of helping others and getting a perspective on life, including the value of education, she went back to Texas. She returned to college and graduated. She worked in direct care services with children in the Texas foster care system. Katharine held that job for five years and decided that she wasn't going to climb the ladder without a master's degree. After receiving her master's degree, she ended up where she is today, as a mental health policy analyst in Austin.

And while she says that statistics were not her thing in school, part of her job requires her to analyze statistics, among many other duties, including interacting with and advocating for the people the organization is serving. "Social services is about people," says Katharine. And with her engaging personality and her ability to forge relationships, she's found a great fit.

Much of Katharine's job involves community engagement. She works with the community, other mental health providers, stakeholders, and those who use the services of mental health providers, including law enforcement and legislators. What she loves about her position is that she is able to create awareness about mental health issues as well as making changes in how those with mental health issues are served and viewed.

Katharine has some advice for those with ADHD. She feels that those with ADHD need to be open to new experiences as well as be willing to explore new opportunities. "I think we can create our own path and our destiny through all our different experiences," says Katharine. "I wouldn't be where I am today without all the barriers and challenges I faced in school." She feels that you figure out what types of things you like, what you can tolerate, and what you're actually good at.

"I never thought I would be working in public policy; it was almost by accident," Katharine says. She was complaining to her former boss about a certain policy, and they both agreed to take the issue to the legislature. "I wouldn't have had that opportunity unless I was open to new experiences and willing to take a risk."

Her other piece of advice is to be comfortable with failing. Maybe what you tried is not meant to be, but it's an opportunity to figure out that next phase in your life. Trying new things keeps a person constantly moving forward. And I can tell you from experience that my parents allowed me to crash and burn a few times. Maybe I had a few crazy ideas, like opening up a mini bike repair shop when I had no experience ever fixing a mini bike. That didn't last long, as you might imagine. But it provided an opportunity for me to evaluate my own capabilities and attempt to learn a new skill.

Katharine also advises that once you figure out how you do things and what you love, you should make sure to advocate for yourself. If you are working for someone else, make sure you and your employer try to develop a mutual understanding as to how you operate. If you don't feel comfortable disclosing that you have ADHD, try to have a conversation with your boss to let her understand how you complete certain projects. Maybe you won't come right out and say, "Hey, I have ADHD," but in my experience, most understanding bosses are more concerned about the successful completion of a project, rather than how it happened.

In the next chapter, I discuss the challenges I had growing up as an ADHD kid and the gifts I ultimately found I had as I entered the working world. As you'll see, I had a need to reinvent myself every decade to keep my interest up. And because I didn't go to school for anything specific, I had to find my way in careers that I could jump into headfirst and that I could teach myself how to be good at. Not one of the careers or businesses I talk about in the coming pages did I ever have any formal education for. And I feel that's a good thing.

the ritalin kid

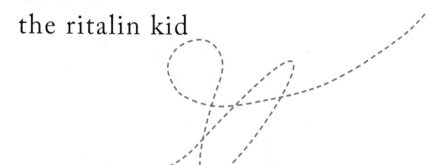

It was probably the day I ran right through the
front storm door of my parents' house that my mother knew I
might be a little different. I was six years old, and with glass and
blood all over the front steps, my mother decided it was time to
have a professional determine whether I might be a bit hyperactive.

I had been sick for over a week, and my mother finally let
me go out and play. As with most kids and adults with ADHD, I
sometimes forgot the details in my quest for the end product. In
this case, in all my excitement, I forgot to hit the door latch before
trying to go through the door. I missed that part. Instead of exiting
the home in a more traditional manner, I went right through the
glass and tumbled down six stairs before landing on the front walk-
way. I had what seemed like hundreds of little cuts all over my body.
Miraculously, my head and all my limbs were still attached. I think
my father still tells this story to his friends.

The next morning our neighbor pulled into the driveway in
her 1970s blue Chevy station wagon to pick up the neighborhood
kids for kindergarten. It was a bright sunny day, and my mother was
more than happy to parade me around with the endless bandages
all over my body to show off how "talented" I was. At this point, she

probably just thought I had a behavior issue—that's the way she decided to deal with me, at least in terms of this episode.

Back in those days, one of the only treatments for kids like me was medication. In my case, it was Ritalin. That, coupled with a child psychologist who to this day kind of freaks me out when I think of sitting with him, was how my parents tried to make me like the other kids. Can't say now it was too effective.

Anyway, when I got really out of control, my mother used to bring me in the bathroom, make me lean over the tub, and spank me. While I was down there, she would shove another Ritalin in my mouth like it was candy. Once again, not sure it really worked. And I'm confident that was not how the drug was prescribed.

My mother passed away before my wife and I had our first and only child. And as we see some of the same traits in Junior—and, sometimes, to a greater degree—I can't help but think my mother is somewhere up there laughing at me (and occasionally with me). And while I love my son with everything I have, I can now see—at least somewhat—what my mother went through with me.

School was a constant struggle, with years of poor grades and the teachers and others trying to figure me out, to no avail. From what I remember, elementary school was not so bad, but when I arrived in what they called junior high school at the time, it was clear I learned differently and was even placed in a special education class. I went to work one afternoon a week at a gas station during class as part of a special program, apparently because the school administrators thought I could benefit from a preview of what I'd be doing for the rest of my life.

After barely making it out of the eighth grade, I went to the vocational school instead of the high school in my town. I thought it might be an easier ride, and for the most part, it was easier than if I had gone to a traditional high school. Until my first year when they kept me back and I had to attend summer school. Okay, maybe I miscalculated. Maybe it wasn't so easy.

High school got so bad for me that there were times I forgot which class I needed to go to. In a vocational school, you go to shop one week and classroom or academics the next week, alternating between the trades and class time. Between that type of schedule and, of course, blowing off school occasionally, there were a handful of times when I had no idea where my class was and ended up wandering around my high school. How I managed to get out of high school on time is probably a miracle in the eyes of the educational system.

At that point, I wanted nothing to do with education and decided to pass on college. Looking back, that was a good move. I would have crashed and burned in record time had I gone to college right out of high school. And quite a few I spoke with for this book had the same experience, doing very poorly in their first year at college.

 ## MY DISTINGUISHED DISHWASHING CAREER

When I was in high school at sixteen years old, I got my first legitimate job. I say "legitimate" because before that, when I was fourteen to fifteen years old, I worked for a contractor as a helper. He paid me under the table. When he started a new job on a house, he would drop me off there for the day and have me demolish whatever room he was working on. On many occasions, I would have to demolish an entire kitchen. Now I don't care who you are, but being fourteen years old and taking a sledgehammer to a kitchen, bringing it right down to the studs, is more fun than you'll ever have. And I might not have known it at the time, but I think it may have been good therapy for my hyperactivity. Because, as I mentioned, I hated traditional therapy.

But at sixteen, I was washing dishes at a restaurant in town called Brigham's. Yes, washing dishes. Given my track record in school over the years, this might have been the last and only stop on a long career as a clean dish technician. Brigham's was a Boston tradition and made just about the best ice cream in the country. During that time, there was one on nearly every corner in greater Boston. Anyone who has ever spent any time in Boston knows all about Brigham's. Aside from selling ice cream, the chain was known for quick-service food, such as burgers, sandwiches, grilled cheese, and breakfast.

After washing dishes for a while, I was asked to work the grill, and for some reason unknown to the ADHD world, this was a great match for my personality. A restaurant kitchen could be an utter disaster for someone with ADHD, as you might imagine. Not quite sure why, but I could quickly run circles around most people in the kitchen. And I could keep all the orders in my head and have them come out of the kitchen on time and in order. Not every time, but, I have to say, I was pretty good on the grill. I remember on one occasion, when it was incredibly busy, I threw the manager out of the kitchen as she tried to help me. She was only getting in the way. I got the death stare, but customers got their food and I didn't get fired. I was hyperfocusing and multitasking at the same time, and she was throwing me off. I went on to cook for several years after that and was tapped to help open their largest store ever, pretty much running the kitchen.

Now you would think an ADHD kid in the kitchen would be an absolute disaster. And, yes, there were times when it looked like an episode of *The Lucy Show*, but most days were in order, and there were many days when I was better off in the kitchen all by myself.

After barely graduating from high school, I ended up working a couple awful jobs in welding. I hated that, and three years spent becoming a certified welder in high school went down the drain in about six months as I realized the job wasn't for me. I went back to Brigham's and eventually became a manager. Yeah, I had to flip a lot of burgers and make a ton of milk shakes, but eventually I was given some responsibility.

 BEING SELF-EMPLOYED

Many ADHDers become self-employed. Some make it big, and others struggle with one scheme after the next. For me, it has been a combination of both.

Many people with ADHD do not like authority, myself included. They're also somewhat impatient. That's why you see many of us drop out of school and start our own businesses. I have started or taken over a number of businesses, including a karate studio, a restaurant, and, as I mentioned, a PR firm. Sounds pretty ADHD, huh? Three completely different types of businesses.

All had their ups and downs, but at the end of the day, I was in control—something, again, that ADHD folks crave. For the most part, no one told me what to do, and if I had a customer I felt was not a good fit for me, I took care of the situation. To this day, I still stick to that way of doing business. Nothing stresses me out more than having a client who is not a good fit. I am fortunate enough at this stage of the game to able to cut them loose if they become a source of stress for me and my staff.

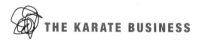 **THE KARATE BUSINESS**

I was kind of geeky growing up. I managed to have a number of friends, but I was always looking to up my stature in the popularity department. I don't know about other ADHD folks, but recognition is something many of us crave to keep us motivated. That's why I think public relations was a good career move for me. Getting on TV was the ultimate high.

As I weaved my way into new groups of friends, my sometimes-too-enthusiastic efforts also got me closer to other kids who didn't really appreciate the way I operated. And the beatings commenced. Eventually, I got tired of getting my ass kicked, and I got tired of not being someone others looked up to. So I decided to take karate. It didn't give me the instant results I wanted, and I didn't follow through with it (big surprise there), but my interest lingered, and I ended up picking it up again after high school.

At that point, I joined a karate and kickboxing school in the next town, and this time, I stuck with it. I fell in love with the martial arts. It made me feel great; I got good at it; it gave me focus; and I was well on my way to becoming a black belt. After a number of years, I passed my first black belt test. I went from a geeky kid with a Dutch boy haircut to a black belt.

After teaching at the school for a couple of years, I tested for my second-degree black belt and earned that rank as well. I really got into the martial arts, studying judo and aikido at other schools. Once again, it made me feel good, confident, and gave me focus—something I needed at the time.

The karate school was the first of my "real" businesses. When I reached my second-degree black belt, a school came up for sale, as the owner wanted out. The school was practically handed to me without many strings. Because I so desperately wanted to create and be in charge of my own venture, I jumped at the chance, and I was in business in no time. I'll preface the rest of this story by saying, there's no better way to learn about business than going in and out of business in less than one year.

I got a lawyer, looked over the books as best I knew how to, and, in no time, I was the proud owner of a karate school. As naive as I was, initially I was also a very happy guy, having achieved a huge milestone in my life: I was truly self-employed.

I mentioned that I consulted a lawyer and looked over the books. My lawyer was a family friend whose specialty was criminal law—not contract law. I got frustrated with him very quickly, and in a short time discounted his advice (remember what I said about ADHD people being quick to discount the advice of authority figures). I was given the books by the current owner, and, at least on paper, the business had a fair amount of receivables that were owed to the business. That ended up not being accurate, and I ended up collecting about $900 when I took over the place. OK, not such a good start, but I was in charge. And, did I mention, I owned my own business?!

Business took off, and for several months, membership was increasing and I was living the dream. I was even teaching Hell's Angels how to kickbox. Imagine a geeky, skinny kid with few friends going on to teach tough biker guys. I was certainly proud of myself!

One of the Hell's Angels I taught even ended up in a very successful movie called *A Bronx Tale* that featured Robert DeNiro. If you have ever seen the movie, you will no doubt remember that famous bar scene with the bikers and the mob. While the bikers lost in the movie—after all, it was Hollywood—I was still pretty proud that maybe he brought some of the skills he learned at my school to the movie set.

I was operating the karate school in the early 1990s, in the middle of a recession. While I got off to a great start, the business quickly took a turn for the worse. I found myself behind on rent and all my other obligations. I tried to get out of my contract with the franchisor, but he wouldn't have anything to do with it. So I packed up the place and shut it down.

Many folks with ADHD will tell you that when they do make a decision, they can execute it in no time. And that's exactly what I did. That school was empty within a couple hours. And what's even stranger is that I felt great about it.

One common trait among people with ADHD is the inability to make a decision. However, once the decision is made, it's like a huge weight is lifted off their shoulders. The one bad thing about this is sometimes a decision can be knee-jerk and backfire. In this case, my decision was totally knee-jerk, but luckily it was the right move. The franchisor ended up going down the toilet himself a couple years later, and I was glad I didn't go with him.

I have to say, as a general comment, I rarely regret a decision. I have a great gut instincts most of the time. Either that or I am very good at moving on and being comfortable with my decisions.

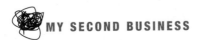 ## MY SECOND BUSINESS

I went back to the restaurant business after shutting down the karate school. After being a manager for a few years in different locations, I was able to purchase a Brigham's franchise. I was dying to be my own boss and now was my chance. You could say I was hyperfocused on being my own boss. Whatever it was, I made it happen because I was determined to do so.

I used savings bonds that had been set aside for college in part to buy the place. My father hesitated slightly but, in the end, he let me do it because it was my money, my college track record was non-existent, and I guess he felt I needed to find my own way. And that was a great trait of my father's: He let me figure things out, instead of protecting me all the time from myself.

It was at about this time in my life that I decided I wasn't going to be that unfocused ADHD kid any longer. I became entirely driven to build this business up and make up for the train wreck that was my past several years of school and work.

The store I took over was also a train wreck. It was owned by an older man who had a stroke right in the store while he was working. I think he worked himself to death.

The store was one of the company's older franchises, and it hadn't been updated in decades. Sales were very low, and it was a massive undertaking to get the business back on track. Luckily, what I soon realized was that this was my wheelhouse. I had an open field to make this business my own and turn it around. From day one, sales started to go up.

I cleaned the place up, eventually remodeling the store, raising prices, and hyperfocusing on great customer service. Yes, I said "raising prices." The prices on the menus were way below what they should have been. In fact, the previous owner's son told me that his father priced items a certain way so they would not have to make changes. *Huh??* I thought that was absurd.

I was hesitant to raise prices at first, but did it anyway, and I have to say that I did not get much negative feedback. Raising prices and raising the customer experience went hand in hand, and it was a risk that paid off well. It was very rare that I had a week when sales and the customer count were down over the previous year. And I have to say that I credit the high energy that came with my ADHD for the overall customer experience in that store.

I knew that no one wants to go into a store and be waited on by a miserable person. You want someone behind that counter who has energy and a passion for what he does—even if it's scooping ice cream. I believe that my high-energy, ADHD style of dealing with customers was a huge marketing tool. I taught all my employees to treat customers the same way: with smiles, high energy, a happy demeanor, and giving them what they want. Just this type of customer interaction alone with no advertising or outside marketing grew sales dramatically.

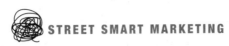 STREET SMART MARKETING

When I began writing this book, I was still running my PR and video marketing firm. It was always called David A. Greenwood and Associates because, quite frankly, it was easier for me to stay a sole proprietor than to create a corporation. I like things to be simple, and putting checks in the bank, at least in my mind, was much easier if the structure of my business stayed simple as well.

In 2014, I changed the name of my company to Street Smart PR/Video to reflect what I felt was my brand—being street smart. In my business, I like to create and execute ideas fast.

And that's exactly what I did in the restaurant. Little did I know back then that I had a mind for marketing and public relations. It was more PR that drove sales than traditional marketing. When I had an idea, I acted on it, and, within record time, we were executing new marketing and PR ideas.

It got to the point, however, that I enjoyed working *on* the business rather than *in* the business, which I guess is a good thing. The problem with that boiled down to a few factors. First, with franchise fees and all the other expenses, it wasn't an operation that you could run without being in the business. You would spend way too much on payroll. Second, the economy was doing very well, and my store was in one of the wealthiest communities in the state, which meant getting help for that type of business became more of a challenge. Because I had trouble getting help, the stress mounted, and there were more than a handful of days when I worked short-handed. And guess what? The public doesn't care if you don't have enough help. You get treated poorly; you get pissed off; and it starts a vicious circle of unhappiness. And when many ADHD folks are unhappy, we walk.

And that's what I did, with a strategy, of course. I couldn't just lock the doors. But one day I did. I had worked two days without much help. In the afternoons in the winter, I could actually tend to the store by myself for a few hours while business was slow. One of those days I started to feel my nose getting wet. I realized that I was getting a nosebleed. Thank God no one was in the store, and I was able to lock the door. I had a nosebleed like you've never seen before. I sat down on the dish room floor until it stopped. Thinking back, that could have been where they found my body if it was something worse, but I chalked it up to stress. And that was it—I sold the place back to the company and walked away.

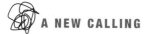 **A NEW CALLING**

I took about six months off after getting rid of the restaurant. I had put aside some money, but it was drying up faster than I had planned. I tried to start my own small PR business but realized very quickly that my experience promoting my store was not nearly enough to get any clients. That was a bit of naive thinking on my part.

During that time, I was volunteering for Special Olympics in my area, helping with PR for about fifteen towns. I was helping what they called an area manager, who, at the time, seemed like just a very nice semiretired man. It was a chance to hone my PR skills without going back to school. I did that for several months and saw a job posting for the Special Olympics PR director for the state of Massachusetts. I initially ignored the job posting because I didn't think I was qualified enough, but after seeing the job posting come up multiple times, I figured I would give it a shot. And I got the job.

It worked out great for both Special Olympics and me. I got some amazing high-profile experience working for such a well-known organization, and I brought a nontraditional approach to getting media coverage to the organization. Oftentimes, I was working with several TV cameras and crews at one time and seeing my work pay off in the form of TV coverage. It was a high I cannot describe. And for this ADHD guy, it was clearly that dopamine my brain needed. I remember our CEO talking after our largest event of the year, the Summer Games held in Boston. He was thanking the staff for a great job, but he also singled me out. I had been there less than a year, and he praised me in front of the entire staff for getting the most press coverage he had ever seen. More dopamine, please. I was on another high.

My work did not go unnoticed, and I was soon tapped to help out with national events for Special Olympics. *Wow, I was scooping ice cream and mopping floors two years ago,* I thought to myself.

I was good at what I did, and my work was noticed by the communications people at the world headquarters in Washington, DC. They asked me to work on a forty-city tour with the Olympic gymnasts who were coming back from the Sydney Olympics. A partnership was formed with Special Olympics, and in each city of the tour, Special Olympics athletes did a routine with the Olympic gymnasts in a stadium. It was a great chance to get into the big-time in public relations and make some huge connections.

We kicked off the tour in Reno, Nevada. At a rehearsal, I was introduced to one of the coaches, who just happened to be from Massachusetts, where I lived. We talked for quite a while about Boston and many other things about living in the Bay State. About an hour later, I was talking to one of the sports anchors from NBC Sports who was covering the tour and doing an hour-long special on the show. I told her I was from Massachusetts, and then she mentioned that the coach was from Massachusetts as well. I went back over to him, completely forgetting our previous conversation and told him that "the woman from NBC Sports told me you were from Massachusetts."

He looked at me and, as you might expect, thought I was nuts. "Didn't we just have this conversation?" I was horrified, to say the least, and looked like a fool. I was overstimulated, trying to do my job, and working on a world-class sporting event with dozens of professional gymnasts I had seen on TV for years. There were camera crews, staging, lights, and I was in the big-time and had completely forgotten our previous conversation. I'm not sure I was even paying attention when we were having that talk. Now I could have just blamed it on my ADHD and made fun of myself, but I decided to walk away, feeling like a total idiot. Not sure we ever had a meaningful conversation after that day. Hell, I wouldn't remember anyway.

Many people can't remember people's names, and I believe entire books have been written about how to remember names. But this has and continues to be a challenge for me. I don't think I have reintroduced myself to someone after that incident, but I will often forget a person's name at a business networking event. I also do it on the phone to this day, and when I know I have done it, at the end of the conversation I will ask him to spell out his name for me to make sure I have it right. "Let me make sure I have the correct spelling of your name." What I'm actually doing is covering my ass because I most likely forgot his name after five minutes.

But that high-profile experience didn't end there, and I was presented with a challenge like none I had ever faced. Remember the area manager I was volunteering for before I worked at Special Olympics Massachusetts? Well, he had been running a secret fund-raising scam for years, and no one but his daughter knew anything about it. She was involved as well and ultimately did some jail time for her involvement.

He would have volunteers call people and get them to donate money to what they thought was the organization. But, in fact, it was going to a secret bank account and never made it to the organization. He and his daughter falsified bank signature cards and created their own little pipeline of free cash. When they slipped up one day and the police were tipped off, it was discovered that he had raised more than $1 million over the course of a few years.

As the money never went through any official bank account, the organization never saw the money. But it was clearly raised in the name of Special Olympics, and the courts agreed that it was a crime.

Cue the media firestorm.

After months of investigations by police and the district attorney, charges were filed against the man and his daughter. While we had a little time to prepare for this because it was an active investigation, nothing can really get you in the frame of mind to face a wall of TV cameras, flashbulbs, and shouting reporters. You see these scenes on TV, but when they are directed at you, it brings a whole new perspective to being nervous. And the word "nervous" might be just a bit of an understatement. What the hell did I get myself into?

On the day of the arraignment, TV cameras, microphones, and a ton of reporters were just waiting for us as far as my eye could see. I almost felt like passing out from all the stress but channeled my energy into our strategy of answering every single question that was asked of us that we could legally answer. We decided to stay until they had no more questions, treating the reporters as if they were at a press event and not a legal proceeding. We helped them with their reports, and we gave them all the information we possibly could give them. We were not combative, and in the end, they ran out of questions. Our strategy paid off, and within twenty-four hours, the news was gone.

While this news literally spread across the country, we were praised for the way we handled it. There was very little damage to the organization, and for the most part, it was back to business. And, wow, did I find something I was great at. One trait of those with ADHD is that they are good in a crisis. When all hell breaks loose, those with ADHD can actually think more clearly. I learned quite a bit about myself through this experience. I was good in crisis, too.

This type of work really fed my ADHD. It was fast-paced and high energy, and at times, it was full of crisis and quick decision making. And because I had brought a new perspective to the workplace and didn't follow the textbook version of how to do my job, I was able to bring something new and effective to the team I worked with, and also make business decisions that ultimately were successful.

I was eventually promoted to vice president with a responsibility for fund-raising, marketing, and public relations and enjoyed that position until I decided to go back out on my own and start a PR firm. I wasn't doing much PR work in the position of vice president, and after a few years, I realized that I missed it. After my mother passed away, I reflected on what I was doing and made the difficult decision to leave the organization. In 2005, I opened up my small public relations firm. In record time, I used the great contact list I had built up over the years, signed up my first client, and was off and running.

While I may have jumped around careers over the past few decades—a common ADHD trait—I have always believed that you should be interested in what you do for a living. Many ADHDers are serial entrepreneurs and are always on the lookout for the next great thing to help satisfy their needs. In that respect, I am no different from many of the people you'll read about in this book.

Enough about me—let's meet some other entrepreneurs and find out how they made their ADHD work in their favor.

CHAPTER THREE

ADHD adults: who are we?

Why are we unique?

One stereotype image of people with ADHD is that they fly into a meeting, throw a bunch of ideas on the table, and walk out. That might be the impression some have of adults with ADHD, and in many cases, they are spot-on. But others who have ADHD and have built very successful businesses are people who don't think like others. They think outside the box, to use an overused term. They come up with incredible ideas, and they have enthusiasm that many don't have. They also take risks. And, in many cases, that's a good thing. Look at history and you'll see countless examples of progress being made because someone had a great idea and took a risk.

One person you'll meet in this book founded a firm that made its name on creating PR stunts for clients. He credits his ADHD with being able to come up with those ideas and take risks. Many of these risks paid off well for his clients in the form of press coverage and increased awareness.

Let's tackle something right here. In my nonmedical humble opinion, we are not ill, and we are not sick. We don't have an affliction, and we are not disabled. As Lady Gaga says, we were born this way. In fact, most people in this book are happy they have ADHD. They have molded their lives around being just a little different, and many have used their ADHD to leverage fabulous ideas. In my years working with Special Olympics, I was surrounded by individuals with physical and intellectual disabilities. But just like the many amazing people I met there, one thing successful people with ADHD do have in common is that we focus on our abilities. And, if anything, I learned valuable life lessons being around the athletes of Special Olympics and their families. One lesson is very clear: Leverage your abilities. Successful people with ADHD do just that.

Some in the ADHD community focus on what they *can't* do. One promise to you here is that you won't meet any of those people in this book. While many I interviewed for this book, including myself, had some tough years—getting kicked out of school, flunking out of school, misbehaving because we were frustrated in our ability to learn, and ultimately realizing we were down to our last dollar—we found a way to make it work. The professionals I had the great honor of interviewing leveraged their ADHD and found a way to become something. Not everyone is a traditionally "successful" millionaire, but many have defined their own success.

I won't be so naive as to say that we don't have bad days, because everyone with ADHD does. I have days where I just can't get out of my own way. And most of those I interviewed for this book feel the same way. ADHDers all have days where they just wish it was over so they could start fresh the following day. Whether you have ADHD or not, don't we all have days where we just end up getting nothing done? I think so. Every one of us is sometimes guilty of staring out the window, thinking about what we're going to do this weekend, or that next vacation in the Caribbean. We're not so different after all, are we? Or are we?

SO WHAT MAKES ADHD FOLKS UNIQUE?

If you truly are ADHD, then you probably know what you are not good at or you have focused on the negative aspects of being an adult with ADHD. We'll address those negative traits in a minute. But what all of us who have been successful in life want you to focus on is the beauty and positive aspects of ADHD. After all, that's the theme of this book. Let's talk about the advantages of being ADHD. And soon we'll get into how to manage the not-so-positive traits of being an ADHD adult.

we are fun!

Many of us with ADHD have great personalities. We love to talk and have meaningful conversations. And in many cases, we can articulate great thoughts and ideas. I mentioned that when I was at Special Olympics in Massachusetts, I was promoted to the position of vice president, even though I had no college degree. I truly believe that it was in part because I was a very good communicator. I could give a pretty good speech and move people to take action for the organization. If you're not a great communicator in the non-profit world, you'll have a tough time inspiring anyone to help you, to donate, to volunteer, and more. A college degree does not guarantee your ability to be an effective communicator.

On many occasions I would end up in a meeting with very accomplished executives, asking them for money—in some cases, some of the largest banks in the world. I was dealing with major players, and I'm guessing that they thought I had gone to some Ivy League school to become such a good communicator. Little did they know that I was a guy who almost took the five-year plan at a vocational school, majoring in welding. I just always had the knack and the skills to be able to handle myself in front of businesspeople.

Greg McDaniel, who has ADHD and dyslexia, is one of those great communicators I spent time talking with for this book. Greg is a partner in a very successful real estate firm in Danville, California. It wasn't always that way, and in 2008, Greg lost almost everything he had in the market downturn. But Greg clawed his way back due, in part, to his likability and his communication skills. He became relentless at knocking on doors and making cold calls to build his business and get his life back, and that paid off. It was what he was good at, and he used that ADHD trait to leverage his comeback in real estate. He also produces an increasingly popular podcast on real estate and is the head corporate trainer at his brokerage firm. If he were an introvert and didn't know how to communicate, he'd probably be doing very poorly. When I spoke with him via a video chat, he was an incredibly confident young man. He spoke extremely well, and he conveyed trust and likability.

we are creative

As they say in social media lingo, BOOM! Those of us who have ADHD are a creative bunch, and this, by far, is our greatest asset. When I mention creativity, I don't necessarily mean that in terms of art-related skills, although that may certainly be the case. What I am talking about is the ability to come up with great ideas and to innovate. We see the world through a different lens sometimes, and we can come up with ideas that can change a business or change the world. The National Institutes of Health website has a section on ADHD, mainly for children. A symptom of ADHD is daydreaming. Another one is being bored. The site talks about risks as well as symptoms. Yes, being creative and thinking unlike others is a medical symptom, I say with a bit of sarcasm.

Author and creativity expert Sir Ken Robinson puts it best: "Creativity is putting your imagination to work, and it's produced the most extraordinary results in human culture." He goes on to say that he believes creativity is the foundation of human culture. If you want to be inspired about your ability to be creative, hop online, view some of Ken's videos, and read his books.

Some of the people you will meet in the coming chapters have been extremely creative in their lives. From a young man who founded a cricket farm to another young professional who was creating productivity applications at age thirteen, there are countless examples of individuals who sucked at school but came up with great ideas that are now making them very successful.

we are willing to take risks

I certainly don't know for sure, but my great-great uncle Chester Greenwood might have had ADHD, if the term existed in the 1800s. Chester was the inventor of the earmuff. He dropped out of elementary school and built quite an enterprise. He invented the earmuff in 1873 after ice-skating. His ears were freezing so, being innovative, he came up with the idea of attaching fur together with bailing wire. His grandmother helped him by sewing the fur together, and the earmuff was born. Chester went on to invent many other items, including a spring-tooth rake and an airplane shock absorber, which is a predecessor to the airplane landing gear of today. Chester took a risk by dropping out of grammar school and putting his ideas into action. It paid off. By the early 1900s his company was producing over 300,000 pairs of earmuffs each year. Again, I have no idea if Chester would have been diagnosed as ADHD, but he did have many of the traits.

More than a handful of those with ADHD have taken big risks not only to enjoy life but to establish a new business or career. Dana Rayburn is an ADHD coach who took the risk of dropping everything and traveling around Europe for a year with her husband.

On the subject of taking risks, she says that many don't always have the full view of their risk in mind. "We don't think it through," she says about those with ADHD. "We jump off the cliff and then build a parachute. And we don't have a realistic view of consequences. Frankly, I love that about me. I love that about my ADD. Sometimes it's gotten me in trouble and put me in precarious situations, but I'm good at creating things on the fly and most of us are."

we can hyperfocus

While not always a good thing, hyperfocus does have its advantages. My son can hyperfocus on a TV show or a video game, which, in my opinion, is not a good thing. But when an adult can use her ability to hyperfocus on a project and produce an incredible result, that is when your ability to lose yourself in a task can become valuable. You see software programmers use hyperfocus to their advantage. And I would argue that many in the programming industry do have some degree of ADHD.

In my world, hyperfocus is one of the keys to getting things done. Call it getting in the zone or whatever you'd like to call it, but my ability to immerse myself in a task such as writing for clients or editing videos is clearly how I get things done and how I do them with quality. If I jump from one thing to the next, I can easily make a mistake. But if I set my mind to hyperfocus on writing, for example, I can plow through a ton of work. In the end, I actually write much better if I can lose myself in the act. In my business, I devote entire days to certain modes of working. On some days, I just write for clients, and on other days, I work on video marketing. Being hyperfocused allows me to immerse myself in those tasks and create much better results. Throw a client in there who is disorganized and late with everything and I have to adjust. But I do my best to get in the zone on particular days.

we have a higher level of awareness

I had the privilege of spending some time with Dr. Edward Hallowell in doing the research for this book. As noted earlier, he has helped countless individuals realize they had some form of ADHD. He's written twenty books on the subject, including the best seller *Driven to Distraction*. Many of those I interviewed for this book referenced his books as tools that helped them understand their ADHD.

Dr. Hallowell is a child and adult psychiatrist and has become a trusted resource for the media on ADHD. He's been featured on *Oprah*, *Good Morning America*, and numerous other shows. He often refers to what we are talking about as ADD, rather than ADHD. But remember, the terminology for Attention Deficit Disorder has been evolving for many years, first from merely "hyperactive" into ADD, and then, more recently, ADHD. The term continues to be debated, but regardless of what we call these traits, we are unique in our own ways.

I asked Dr. Hallowell one very simple question: Why do those with ADHD make great entrepreneurs?

He talks about the type of people who set sail on the *Mayflower* and headed for the New World. What kind of person would get on a boat in the early 1600s, set sail across the ocean to a land where there were no roads or other infrastructure, no government or any known resources? Most likely, those who thought differently, those who were visionary, and those who were dreamers, people who were wildly unrealistic and people who wanted to do it their way.

Dr. Hallowell goes on to explain that these people were also tenacious to the point of being stubborn and explorers at heart. And the overriding reason for all of this is the desire to be free. "People with ADD want to be free," says Dr. Hallowell. "It really comes out of an emotional place where these folks just have a tremendous feeling of 'I want to do it my way, I want to be free, I don't want to take orders, I don't want to be in lockstep, I don't want to work in a group where I have to conform and be on time and dot my i's and cross my t's.'"

Dr. Hallowell mentions at this point that he dislikes both terms—ADD *and* ADHD. "It's a complicated kind of mind and it's full of all these swirling forces. I often say to kids that you have this Ferrari engine for a brain and you have this way powerful mind, with bicycle brakes. A lot of the work is trying to control the power of your mind."

Another powerful analogy Dr. Hallowell uses relates to Niagara Falls. As he points out, "Until you build a hydroelectric plant, it's just a bunch of noise and mist. But when you build that hydroelectric plant, you light up the state of New York."

So what is ADHD? "It's a very overdetermined, complicated, and fascinating condition," says Dr. Hallowell. And, he adds, being an entrepreneur is a logical destination for ADHD adults. But not everyone with ADHD goes out and works for themselves, of course. There are other occupations that are equally well suited for those with ADHD minds.

High-intensity careers tend to be uncommonly good options for those with ADHD. Dr. Hallowell notes that many brain surgeons have ADHD, and while they may be super-focused in the operating room, they're often not so good with the paperwork after the surgery. He mentions that those with ADHD make good trial attorneys because of the high energy associated with that career. And, for ADHD adults, the Navy SEALs can be heaven, because ADHD people tend to be very good under pressure.

All of this is why you see ADHD people work in jobs and careers that are often long on creativity and short on conformity, long on chances to innovate and short on demands for repetition.

"ADD is just a shorthand for a collection of symptoms—some positive and some negative," says Dr. Hallowell. He feels that the textbooks mostly discuss the negatives, viewing ADHD as a collection of psychopathology. But he and many others feel strongly that it's a combination of positives and negatives.

When discussing risk taking with Dr. Hallowell who, by the way, also has ADHD, he notes, "We are far more captivated by the dream than held back by the danger. The dream is what motivates us. The dangers, we are aware of but we don't let them captivate us as they captivate most people." Most people first see the dangers, and then, because something may be unrealistic, many of those without ADHD don't move forward. "'Unrealistic' is not in our vocabulary. We're all about go for the gold and damn the torpedoes, full speed ahead."

Dr. Hallowell cautions me that, in many cases, risk taking may lead to trouble because we disregard the danger of taking a risk. "We love pursuing the goal. We're not so concerned about winning the prize. And most of us with ADD are never satisfied."

we focus on our strengths

If you have read any other books about ADHD, you may have read the analogy of the hunters and the gatherers. Dr. Hallowell also alludes to this concept. Back in prehistoric times, there were both types of people on earth. Many experts and researchers believe that those who hunted over ten thousand years ago exhibited many of the characteristics of those with ADHD: They were impulsive risk-takers, and they thrived on crises and situations that demanded problem solving. There has even been research led by anthropology graduate student, Dan Eisenberg of Northwestern University in 2008 on existing indigenous tribes in Kenya that has supported this theory.

The individuals who opted to live out in the open as nomads, as opposed to in more settled populations, based in caves, leveraged their abilities to gather and protect their food sources as well as their families. They also appeared to be in better health and better nourished. The evidence lies in a certain dopamine receptor gene, called the DRD4/7R. Those who had it and lived out in the wilderness were well nourished while the people who also had it and lived in settled populations were not so healthy.

The problem in schools and in many doctors' offices now is that we view these traits as negative, and in many cases are told that they constitute a disability. Many doctors are more likely to diagnose and treat—often with medication—a "disability" than look at the nuanced relationship between personality and what might otherwise be considered a constellation of maladaptive traits.

Risk taking may have led our ancestors out of caves and onto the plains, but another ADHD trait helped them develop the hunting skills that enabled them to provide for their families. Say what you will about daydreaming, but it's one of those ADHD traits that has allowed us to come up with great ideas for tens of thousands of years. And these days, if daydreaming doesn't get in the way of doing your job or fulfilling the responsibilities you have committed to, it continues to be a great way to innovate.

Daydreaming leads to ideas, and ideas lead to innovation. But first you need to learn about your ADHD and build a solid foundation. Having a solid footing will enable you to leverage your ADHD for good. Not having your life somewhat in order will just cause you to continue to stare out that window with no results. Brendan Mahan, an ADHD coach in Massachusetts, says you have to know about your own ADHD and also learn how ADHD works so you can better understand how your personal type of ADHD affects you.

Brendan uses this example: "Knowing that your ADHD makes it hard for you to get to places on time is one thing. Understanding why is another. It could be that you're late because you get lost in tasks and often don't realize how long it takes you to get things done. That's connected to poor time awareness, a challenge common to ADHD. It might also be that you're often late because your ADHD hinders your ability to plan and prioritize. Maybe you think you're leaving yourself enough time—you have a meeting at 1:30 p.m., it takes a half hour to drive there, so you leave at 1:00 p.m. But you fail to factor in the possibility that there might be traffic, or how long it takes to find a parking place, or the time it takes to walk from the parking lot to the building your meeting is in. The better we understand how our personal version of ADHD affects us, the more effectively we can use strategies and interventions to help manage it."

He is also very adamant about making sure those with ADHD play to their strengths: "There are strengths that come with ADHD; there are weaknesses, too, but there are strengths." Creativity and excitement are two that readily come to mind for Brendan. He points out the advantage of seeing issues in a different way. Brendan feels that those with ADHD end up making connections where other people don't see them because the ADHD brain files things in different spots, connecting things in different ways than they are connected in everyone else's brain.

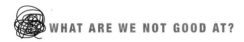 **WHAT ARE WE NOT GOOD AT?**

There are positives and negatives with ADHD. I focus mostly on the positives here, but knowing the negative manifestations of your ADHD can help you strengthen the positives. Much of this book is spent offering you real-world techniques on how to turn your negatives into positives. But regardless if you have ADHD or not, as humans we have to realize that there are things in life that we might not be good at. Not everyone with ADHD falls into these traits but these are general observations.

we get distracted easily

You might think it's just your kid who can't pay attention, but we adults may be guilty of that as well. The number of times I'm thinking about something else when someone is talking to me is in the millions. I tend to keep focused on the conversation if the person is saying something interesting, but once the conversation turns to a less engaging topic, the brain of an adult like me with ADHD moves on to something else. More than that, in the age of social media, distractions are hitting us from all angles. Those with ADHD are prone to being thrown off track just by their own unrelated thoughts, but when you add intrusions from blinking and buzzing phones and other distractions like email, forget it. You might be having a conversation or meeting with someone at work, and she says something that causes you to start thinking about another project, or your phone vibrates with a request for an update on another project, and you start to think about that. And off you go.

we procrastinate

My wife jokes that she won't buy me any more Christmas gifts because I never use the ones she gives me. Okay, she's half kidding, but I do have gifts that I have yet to even take out of the box. I have all the items to make beer, including all the pans, tanks, and ingredients. Have I made beer yet? No. Many I spoke with note that this was the most prominent trait with their ADHD. We just have a hard time getting started—for some reason our brain tells us it will take too long to read the instructions and tends to suggest something more easily accessible, even if the long-term reward of finally setting up that home-brewing equipment could be immensely satisfying.

we lack organization

Not everyone who has a huge pile of papers on his desk has ADHD, but it is one of the clearer indications that ADHD might be an issue. Adults with ADHD often fail to set up the proper system for staying on top of things at work and at home, and that leads to being chronically disorganized. We often procrastinate, putting things in the right places but walking away before actually doing what needs to be done, and that leads to larger and larger piles. We may not be hoarders, but we often do have telltale piles of stuff lying around in configurations that may not make any sense to other people.

we are late and we forget

Why is it so difficult for us to maintain an up-to-date calendar and to-do list? This is the first question some ADHD coaches ask a client. And just about all the people I spoke with say that if they don't immediately write something down, it's gone. For some reason, we ADHDers think we will remember something when it's given to us or a thought pops into our heads. I can forget something as I'm walking from the kitchen to the bedroom. And then I wonder what I'm doing in the bedroom. "Why did I walk into the bedroom?" I'll wonder. Others are chronically late. They fail to estimate how long a task will take or how long it takes to get somewhere. And many times they are just wrapped up in something else.

we don't always follow directions

OK, ladies, make your jokes here about men not following directions. Maybe you're right. But many of us don't like to even read the directions to something. We purchase a product—maybe it's a snow blower—and we discard the directions. Many adults with ADHD think, "How hard can it be?" Put some gas in it, pull the starting cord, and start getting rid of the snow, right? But then when we can't get it started, we get pissed off and wonder what's going on. Your spouse may know why: You probably didn't read the directions. This may also lead to a bit of an authority complex. We may not be very good at following directions, and we don't like the authority figures who direct us, so we try to do things are own way. That's why many adults with ADHD work for themselves.

we take the good with the bad

Just because you have any of these characteristics doesn't mean you have ADHD, as it's clinically defined. Diagnosis should be left to a medical professional. However, here's a helpful rule of thumb that may clue you in to whether you just have the kind of problems with focus that plague most of the human population, or something more pervasive that may be called ADHD: Though the criteria change periodically, if you have at least six or seven of the most common symptoms of inattention or hyperactivity, you may be diagnosed with it. And, while you can go on a whole host of websites that detail the kind of symptoms you may have, you should go to the website for the Centers for Disease Control (CDC) or another credible organization (see the resources section at the end of this book). When you have a reasonable idea that you may be an ADHD adult, find a professional in the medical field to get an official diagnosis.

Take a moment to reflect on what we have discussed in this chapter and see how many of these good and bad traits sound like yours. Even make a list. The whole point is to continue to learn about what you are good at and what you might not be so good at. Try something as simple as taking out a legal pad, writing down these things, and reflecting on them. Once you do this, the next chapter will be even more useful for you as we discuss building a solid foundation as an adult with ADHD.

a solid foundation

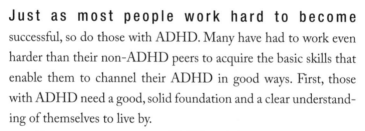

Just as most people work hard to become successful, so do those with ADHD. Many have had to work even harder than their non-ADHD peers to acquire the basic skills that enable them to channel their ADHD in good ways. First, those with ADHD need a good, solid foundation and a clear understanding of themselves to live by.

For you to manage your ADHD and thrive with it, you need to take care of your mind and body and you need to implement certain routines in your daily life. By the same token, you also need to take a personal inventory of yourself. Do you understand your ADHD, and do you have a firm grasp of what is getting in your way? Do you have trouble focusing at work? Do you forget to do important tasks? Do you stay up all night, and are you then tired all day? A solid foundation and an understanding of your ADHD can help you correct the habits that are getting in the way of your success.

Many of us, when left to our own devices, will spin our wheels and chase our tails. While we might have the next huge idea for a business, without a firm foundation on which to leverage our strengths, we will crash and burn. While many of us are great in a crisis, we don't want to live in crisis mode 365 days a year. There's a clear difference between being valuable in a crisis and having your life become one.

If we just get up each day without a plan or an idea of what our day will look like, it is almost certain that it will spin out of control. The same goes for how we live our lives and take care of our mind and body. All successful individuals, whether or not they have ADHD, have taken the steps to implement basic principles in their lives that help them at work, at home, and in life in general.

I spent some time with ADHD and executive function coach Brendan Mahan, who's based in Massachusetts. Brendan works with adults and children with ADHD and has spent quite a bit of time coaching college students with ADHD. Brendan himself was diagnosed with ADHD as an adult, much like many other coaches I interviewed. Brendan counsels college-aged individuals, and he helps them build a foundation so that when they actually get out into the labor market or decide to go into business, if they choose, they have the habits they need to be successful.

As I interviewed Brendan via a video chat, a new heating system was being installed in my office building. The arc welder was positioned right under my office window. The perfect timing and, of course, the perfect position drove me just a little nuts. I've always known that certain sounds bother me. However, I mentioned to Brendan that, at my age, fifty years old, I had just begun to realize that I may have sensory issues. Many with ADHD also exhibit some type of sensitivity to various sounds, feelings, smells, and other stimuli. While what they call "sensory processing disorder" is a separate diagnosis from ADHD, many, including myself, have a low tolerance for certain sounds and other stimuli. This might be one reason a child in a restaurant has a temper tantrum. You might think she is just misbehaving, but what you actually might be witnessing is her inability to handle all the stimulation. Is it ADHD or sensory processing disorder? Some feel the symptoms overlap. Back to the arc welder. I think anyone would have been bothered by the sound, but that hypersensitivity to sounds and other things going on around you really irritates many with ADHD who have concentration issues.

"Wouldn't it have been awesome when we were kids if this stuff was talked about," Brendan says to me. "So much of sensory issues and ADHD—the more you learn about it, the more effectively you can manage it." Brendan goes on to say that the more we know about our particular ADHD traits, the easier it is to adapt to them. Which leads us to learning about ourselves and building a foundation.

Brendan feels there are several things that people with ADHD, regardless of their age, need to build into their life. And, in speaking with others, I have listed a few more. The first thing he feels is an absolute must is getting enough sleep. While eight hours is always ideal, according to most experts, every individual has different needs. Many people do great with six hours of sleep while other people might need nine hours. Brendan also feels strongly that people with ADHD, in particular, need to develop a pattern of sleep; that is, they need to go to bed and wake up at the same time each day. That includes the weekends—which I will confess is a hard thing to become accustomed to. And forget about trying to make up for lost sleep on the weekends. While it may feel great to sleep in, trying to compensate for a sleepless week by staying in bed all weekend doesn't help people with ADHD because it breaks up the pattern they need to develop. "You need to get yourself in the habit of sleeping on a regular schedule and sleeping the right amount," says Brendan. If you don't get enough sleep, your ADHD can actually be much worse the very next day. I can tell you from my own personal experience that if I sleep poorly, it pretty much sets the tone for my entire next day."

My son, who has more energy than anyone I know, has been known to come into our bed in the middle of the night—sometimes around 3 or 4 a.m. His mind is racing so much that he starts to giggle while we are trying to sleep. Couple that with him moving every ten seconds or so and that is a recipe for a bad night's sleep. Some days I can dust myself off, and I'm all right. But on other days, it sets me up for an unproductive day.

Habits are critical to a solid foundation, according to Brendan. "You have to have more good habits than bad habits," he points out. Proper sleep is definitely a good habit, and so are other rituals, such as planning your day ahead of time, and preplanning, like making the kids' lunches the night before and having a game plan before you hit the office. Habits can also be routines you follow every morning. For me it's coffee, shower, and get my son out of bed, fed, and out the door to the bus.

For the days when my wife puts Junior on the bus, I follow roughly the same routine, even though it's not my responsibility to get him on the bus. Brendan also feels it is absolutely worth making time each day for some type of meditation. "I encourage a meditation or mindfulness practice with all my clients and everybody I talk to who has ADHD, because taking time out of your day to slow down and let your brain chill out for a little bit is going to help you fall asleep and help you be more productive. There's all kinds of science and research into the benefits of mindfulness practices and how beneficial they are for productivity and performance and for your brain in general." Many people I spoke to for this book have said that meditation keeps them moving in a forward and positive direction.

Those with ADHD often have racing minds. Many times, we are either thinking a mile a minute about a specific subject, or we are all over the place. Many of us just can't stop. Meditation can help slow the process down and actually provide a little more stability to the brain and our thoughts. An intense and productive creative process, one of the hallmarks of an ADHD adult, can be hugely beneficial, as we've discussed. But if you can't make sense of the thoughts or ideas, they end up as no more than that: thoughts and ideas, with no plan for their execution.

Some with ADHD are introverts while others are more outgoing. But, whatever the case is with you, relationships are particularly important to adults with ADHD. Strong relationships can contribute to that solid foundation we outlined earlier in this chapter. "You've got to have social connections both because you have to have that support but also because we are social animals," says Brendan. "We need people we care about and people who care about us." He goes on to say that if you look at this through the lens of success, the more connections you have, the more opportunity for success you will have. I feel that you need both strong personal and strong professional relationships, people in your life who can make you feel good about yourself instead of making you doubt yourself and your gifts.

Adults with ADHD often have no issue carrying on a conversation—in fact, many of us have a tendency to talk too much at certain times, for example, when we are particularly excited about something or if we are engaged in a conversation where someone is paying a lot of attention to us. In those cases, sometimes we view that as a license to keep on talking. Brendan concurs. I feel that great conversation stimulates the brain and causes us to crave more. As we've discussed, people with ADHD sometimes have issues with impulse control, and that extends to talking with friends, family, and colleagues. It may be challenging to pull back when we're getting such great feelings from an engaging chat with someone whose company we enjoy. It's important for us to surround ourselves with healthy relationships, but also to know when to give others space and back off when necessary.

It's crucial for anyone who is trying to be successful to keep positive people nearby. For someone with ADHD, self-doubt and self-criticism can be huge problems. Whether it's just one bad day filled with a few ADHD-related misses, a string of bad days, or a generalized feeling of shame built up over time, having positive people in your life can bring you back from obsessive self-criticism or possibly depression. We were told for so long growing up to try harder or to pay attention or that we were not good enough, and those negative messages often stick with us.

By surrounding yourself with people you respect and trust, you will also be building a solid support system. A supportive network of close friends and immediate family is critical to a balanced life. If your work life is full of support, but when you get home, your spouse doesn't understand you, that's a problem. And, of course the reverse is true. Having a professional support system, like Brendan, a medical doctor or therapist specializing in ADHD, or the kind of ADHD coaches you meet here, is invaluable. The two coaches I have had over the years have not been ADHD-specific coaches, but we worked very well together. Fit is incredibly important. You may very well decide that a coach might not be enough for you and that there are things in your life that are better discussed with a doctor or therapist. You need to make that decision.

Many, including Brendan, feel that exercise is essentially non-negotiable, and I agree. Peter Shankman, a well-known keynote speaker on the subject of customer service, says that you should not go more than forty-eight hours without some form of exercise. And I feel the same way. After about two days, my mind starts to go places that I don't want it to go, and I need that burst of energy I get from a workout to keep me stable and centered.

There is more than enough science behind the theory that exercise not only helps those with ADHD, but it can also be a primary part of treatment. Boosting dopamine in the brain eases stress, controls anxiety, and improves overall executive function. Regular exercise also helps you sleep better, improves your overall mood and memory, and can be a great way to break up a boring day. And if you eat like a caveman, as I do, then it also helps keep that waistline trim.

EXCUSES

Using your ADHD diagnosis as an excuse will not serve you well. "History is probably the worst offender in these situations," says Dr. Judi Cineas, a licensed clinical social worker in Florida. "Sometimes the person who has been diagnosed will identify as the diagnosis, and that's one of the things I try to break people out of." Mind-set is a major element in creating success, whether you are ADHD or not. And if you blame your ADHD for every little failure or inadequacy in your life, you'll be spinning your wheels until you wake up and realize that what you have can be leveraged.

Recognize that there are tasks you are not good at. Find a way to achieve your goals in spite of these weaknesses, and focus on your strengths. If you can't seem to manage your accounting books or your schedule, hire someone to do it in your business. That's not a new concept. Businesspeople and executives delegate tasks to others all the time. You can't be good at everything, and some of your problems will be directly related to your ADHD. But you are doing yourself a disservice if you blame your ADHD for all your shortcomings.

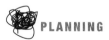

PLANNING

Find a way to plan everything, even if that means writing things down on a legal pad before you begin each new task. In short, make planning part of your life. Oftentimes, when starting a new business, one person does all the work, and maybe that's you right now. To get your new business off the ground, you are doing everything—and that's not sustainable. Dr. Cineas refers to some people with ADHD as "multistarters" because, as most of us know, we try to start many projects as ideas come to us, instead of planning, focusing, and finishing just a few of them. So in some cases, we end up getting very little done. Impulsive behavior has its place, but when trying to start a business or launch an important project for a business, not having some type of plan is a recipe for missed deadlines and a list of unfinished endeavors.

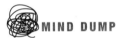

MIND DUMP

Ryan McRae writes the blog *ADHD Nerd*. Ryan coaches, speaks, and has written a few books on ADHD. A basic technique he uses is the "mind dump." When he gets to a point where confusion sets in and he has issues remembering what needs to be done, he performs a mind dump, writing down everything he needs to get done. "I don't care if it's brushing my teeth at night: I just unload it all, because my brain becomes an episode of *Hoarders* and I can't hold onto all of it." Ryan uses an analogy, saying that most people are born with a bulletin board of sorts in their head with pins for different ideas and other things they need to remember. Those with ADHD have the bulletin boards, but no pins. "We slap that piece of paper on the bulletin board, and it just slides down."

Ryan also has a few other tips for building a solid foundation for life as an ADHD adult. He's big on systems: "Develop the systems that work for you, and the minute they stop working, change them." Don't get rid of them, but make small changes to alter them so they work for you. Don't throw the day planner out, just alter the way you use it, advises Ryan.

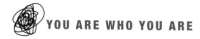

YOU ARE WHO YOU ARE

Forgiveness is critical, according to Ryan. "Just forgive yourself, and do it often. Whether it's hourly, daily, weekly, or whatever it is. Because we fight a really hard battle, because we don't live in a world of artists, we live in a world of architectures." He goes on to say that, for the most part, we live in a world of boundaries and rules, and for many of us, it's a hard way to live. "Give yourself some grace."

Ryan also suggests getting rid of any shame you carry as an adult with ADHD. Having a solid foundation enables you to be comfortable with who you are. "Shame is ADHD and anxiety's fuel, and [they both] just thrive on it. We always want to [believe] that we are better, and shame always tells us we're not better at all. So our ADHD is on a treadmill, and [we] can't get off it." Eventually, Ryan says, because of that, our decision fatigue and our creativity suffer because we feel this way. For those of us with ADHD, that's one of the most toxic things we can do to ourselves. Accepting ourselves leads to accepting our limitations.

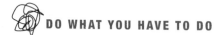

DO WHAT YOU HAVE TO DO

Building a solid foundation means doing what you have to do to become a productive and successful individual. For some people, medication may be necessary.

Although I believe that our society is overmedicated and some doctors are too willing to pull out a prescription pad and start writing, it would be wrong not to acknowledge the beneficial effect medication can have on some people. Every brain is different, and all the circumstances that make up our lives are different. So for all the doctors reading this right now, there are people who need medication and should be using it. If you have ADHD and are struggling to function on a day-to-day basis, talk to your doctor about your options. You may decide that medication is the right strategy for you.

Eric Tivers, LCSW, runs Tivers Clinical Specialties, PC, based in Illinois, and produces the popular online podcast *ADHD reWired*. He works with both ADHD patients and those on the autism spectrum. And he believes that medication does have its place in managing ADHD. Eric is pro-medication, and he believes it can have an enormous beneficial impact in managing your ADHD and your life. "It doesn't work for everybody," he cautions, however. "And for some, the side effects are intolerable," says Eric.

Eric suggests trying medication, if you think you need it. "Really try medication, and try many medications and really give it a marathon of a trial."

But Eric and many others agree that you cannot rely on medication alone to solve all your attention and distraction problems in life. You have to have that solid foundation in your life to survive and thrive with ADHD as an adult. Realize that you are not inherently lazy and that you can leverage your ADHD to make great things happen in your life and career. You can be super-productive with ADHD if you take a holistic approach and manage it from all angles.

"Everything that's not directly related to productivity actually helps productivity," says Eric. It's the quality of sleep and getting enough sleep. It's exercise and also making time for play; it's effectively managing stress through the strategies that work for you. He says that these types of self-care techniques really help an adult with ADHD move forward and feel good. He calls it "energy management" rather than "time management." "Our brain has some challenges so we need to do everything possible to optimize how our brain is functioning."

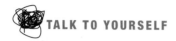**TALK TO YOURSELF**

We've all been caught talking to ourselves, but are we saying the right things?

Chris Berlow is the coauthor of the book *You Have Infinite Power* and a personal empowerment expert. In the interest of full disclosure, I have worked with him over the years in my business.

When Chris coaches an individual, he first tries to help that person identify her limiting beliefs. He works with that person to figure out why she is stuck and helps her think beyond those limiting thoughts. From there he coaches her to understand that she can choose her own thoughts. Having a coach or mentor remind you that your thoughts mean something is a great way to incorporate positive support into how you talk to yourself.

When he conducts programs with his partners for companies and other organizations, Chris says, they ask people what their biggest takeaway was from the program, and more often than not, it was that they really did have the ability to choose their own thoughts. "When you can control your thoughts, you can control your life, and that's true power," says Chris.

To change your limiting thoughts and beliefs, Chris recommends asking yourself this: What is the biggest negative thought trend that you have? For this exercise, come up with three of them. Maybe think back to those report cards you came home with, the ones peppered with criticism from teachers that filled you with shame. Or, if you weren't ashamed of your report cards, it's still likely that many of your negative thoughts stem from your upbringing. For example, many of us grew up at a time when even the term ADHD was nonexistent. Educators and others didn't know what to do with us. We were labeled "problem children" and were ultimately punished by our parents for the things ADHD caused us to do or not to do. Rather than offering support, maybe your father shouted,

"Just try harder" or "Why are you so bad at math?" And maybe we did try harder and got nowhere and still got no support. You may have come to the conclusion that you are just not good at math.

I was never especially fond of sports. When we played kickball, everyone moved closer when it was my turn to kick, because they knew I could not kick the ball very far. I tried out for Little League only to be repeatedly turned away. I told myself I was simply not good at sports. But then I found karate and became a second-degree black belt. I actually did have athletic ability, but I had always told myself that I didn't.

Chris uses the example of a person who wants to get healthy and start exercising. But then that guy tells himself that he is too old, he doesn't have the time, and he doesn't know how to exercise. Chris works with him to find that common thread of negative beliefs, and together they figure out a way to counter those limiting beliefs.

Chris suggests creating an empowering statement that helps get rid of the negative talk and turns your thoughts into positive actions. What is the positive outcome you want out of these thoughts? You want to create a habit of empowering and positive thoughts going through your head, instead of an instinctual negative thought pattern.

Recite your empowering statements five times in the morning and five times in the evening. One person I interviewed for this book gets up every morning, puts his feet on the floor, and says, "It's going to be a amazing day!" Eventually you will believe it, and you will change negative thoughts into positive ones. Don't discount this advice: It works. Reconditioning your mind requires repetition—it's not just a one-time thing.

In short: Go to the gym; eat right; clear your mind periodically; get rid of negative thoughts; build a great support system; and know that you can be even more productive than the kid who sat next to you in elementary school, always did his homework, and got straight A's.

Most super-successful people, regardless of whether or not they have ADHD, have built certain principles and systems into their lives. And those of us with ADHD have to absolutely ensure we have a great foundation to build on, or we can crash and burn in no time.

mind and body

Numerous studies confirm that taking care of your mind and your body is critical in managing and thriving with ADHD. Most people I interviewed for this book stated that exercise and proper amounts of sleep were the two top ways they manage their ADHD. In some cases, these behaviors enabled them to get off medication.

If I don't get to the gym at least every two days, my mind starts to wander and my energy levels take a huge nosedive. Sleep is also vital to those with ADHD. A fresh mind sets your day up for success. But there are additional ways of addressing the mental and physical components of ADHD that have worked for the other people I interviewed for this book.

Carlos Zapata has built a successful investment management company in California. Born in Lima, Peru, he had very frequent suspensions from school, flunked many of his classes, and spent most of his summers in summer school. He moved with his family to the United States halfway through his senior year in high school. When he arrived in California, he was enrolled in a private Catholic high school, and was suspended in his first week. "Growing up, it seemed like everything I did or everything I said, whether it was at school or at home would very easily get me into trouble," says Carlos. "I was very hyperactive, and I was always looking for ways to counteract my hyperactivity, and that brought me quite a bit of trouble, both in school and at home."

His father was a physician, but this was back in the days when many youngsters were just classified as hyperactive, or "problem," children, rather than ADHD. Like many ADHDers, he went undiagnosed until his mid-thirties.

Luckily for Carlos, his school had many different sports programs. And in a country where soccer is almost a religion, he was fortunate that his school offered an array of other sports programs to choose from, including basketball, baseball, and surfing. "I would sign up for absolutely everything the school offered," says Carlos. That kept him out of trouble at school and at home. By participating in these athletic activities every day after school, he could release his energy and hyperactivity. And once he got home, he would feel much more calm, relaxed, and even focused.

"If my mother had any chores for me to do or wanted me to do a particular school project, then I was a lot more focused to embark on requests that she needed me to do. But that was only because I was able to release all that built-up energy I had inside." Whenever that wasn't the case, he would always get in trouble. But most days, he was able to control his ADHD by being heavily involved in sports.

Carlos also believes that growing up with ADHD and having that constant flow of negativity in the form of people, teachers, and others telling him he's wasn't good enough or needed to try harder made him part of who he is today, a successful entrepreneur. He's not afraid of making mistakes, he says, at his age. "I think it has made me much more of a risk-taker in life because of not fearing failure."

Carlos now takes part in many outdoor activities; one of his favorites is road cycling. He sometimes spends up to three hours on his bike, coming back extremely focused and relaxed. And his use of the word "relaxed" is something only an ADHD person can relate to: "When I say I am relaxed after, for example, three hours of riding my bicycle, I am relaxed in a sense I don't feel like I'm coming out of my skin anymore, that I need to run in a thousand different directions at a thousand miles per hour." He feels entirely focused.

While studying for his master's degree, Carlos would go out and bike at least fifty miles in a day. Carlos says that others might need to take a nap after riding fifty to sixty miles, but not him. He would get back and be ready to tackle his assignments. Rigorous exercise, such as bicycling for two or three hours, actually relaxes him and sets him up to be incredibly focused.

Carlos recently sold his investment business and started a new one that focuses more on institutional clients. At the time we spoke, he was incredibly busy and was having difficulty finding the time he wanted to dedicate to his outdoor activities. He had made the shift to taking medication, when necessary, and still got out on his bike whenever he could. But the demands of his business caused him to make a choice to take medication, as needed.

His goal is to once again get off the medication, and he's working toward that every day. Many others I spoke to said that, when needed, they do take some form of medication. When our best efforts to manage our ADHD through exercise and other natural efforts take a backseat to life and the real world, medication may help.

Dr. Jose Colon is a sleep-disorder specialist, based in Florida, and he has ADHD. Dr. Colon is also a fan of that forty-eight-hour exercise rule. "I never go two days in a row without exercising because two days in a row can easily turn into two weeks and two weeks can turn into two months," he says. Dr. Colon is a lifelong fan of exercise, who played football while in school and has received a lot of benefit from physical activity.

Dr. Colon's advice is to fit in some kind of physical activity, even if it's not a full-fledged workout, at least every two days. Even a walk after dinner can clear your mind and improve focus if your schedule is too busy. He's a big fan of the Fitbit™ and other fitness trackers that you place on your wrist like a watch. These products measure your daily activity, including your sleep on some models. He also suggests trying to incorporate some high-intensity workouts. "You don't have to suddenly become a sprinter," he says, but when you're doing a jog around the lake, you can incorporate jumping jacks and push-ups, a couple sprints, and incorporate things that increase your heart rate. That's a great way to keep your workouts challenging and engaging.

"Sometimes when I go to the gym I'm just lifting weights; that's good for you." But he also suggests kicking it up a notch by doing some burpees in between lifting weights, as well as other high-intensity activities that get the heart rate up.

And while this may seem inspiring at best and intimidating at worst, it does make sense, even if you are a stranger to exercising on a regular basis. If you want to get a great introduction to exercise and some outside perspective on setting up a routine that you'll want to follow, consider talking to a personal trainer or another fitness professional. A trainer can teach you how to do different exercises correctly, and how to use the different machinery at the gym, if that's what interests you. Hurting yourself the first day in the gym will only deter you from ever going back.

So what does exercise actually do for you? You may be familiar, at least in passing, with the words "dopamine" and "endorphins." There has been plenty of research to suggest that the ADHD brain lacks the proper amounts of dopamine, a neurotransmitter that helps support the transmission of signals to the brain. Exercise and physical activity have been shown to increase dopamine in the body. When dopamine gets into the frontal cortex of the brain, it allows us to think more clearly. In essence, it can control the flow of information or, in the case of someone with ADHD, the lack of flow.

ADHD medication works to increase the amount of dopamine in the body. But, while exercise has a similar effect, it has many additional benefits: It can also help get you in shape and lose weight, not to mention the satisfaction that comes with successfully completing a difficult task like riding your bike over fifty miles at a time. Exercise will achieve many things in your life and can add to your confidence and clear your mind.

Another thing that researchers have discovered is that exercise increases the amount of brain-derived neurotrophic factor, or what they refer to as BDNF, a protein in the body that has been known to promote healthy nerve cells. Researchers have shown that increased levels of BDNF can increase memory and overall mental functioning. One study, in particular, by researchers at the University of Pittsburgh, states that exercise increases the size of the hippocampus, which produces BDNF. The study also supports the hypothesis that fitness protects against what is called hippocampal volume loss. So, as you get older, exercise is especially important.

A positive self-image is crucial as well, and something ADHD adults often struggle with. Years of people telling us we can do better or that we are not good enough may come back to haunt us. And because many of us have difficulty with authority, when someone criticizes our work, we can get very aggravated and feel as if we aren't good enough. In some cases, we quit and move on. Regular physical activity helps counter that feeling of inadequacy. Our minds feel better; we feel more confident about our bodies; and our self-esteem goes up. Maybe you're a little tired after leaving the gym, but you can't tell me that you don't feel better about yourself.

SLEEP

As I mentioned, Dr. Colon is a sleep-disorder specialist who treats both adults and children. Just about every ADHD coach or other professional I talked to stated that a good night's sleep was absolutely critical to managing ADHD. Most listed it as their number one piece of advice.

Sleep helps your mind and body heal. Dr. Colon states that, when you sleep, you replenish your body's neurotransmitters that have been depleted throughout the day. And as we discussed above, those neurotransmitters help carry signals through the brain. If you do not regenerate those neurotransmitters with a good night's sleep, that's probably the reason you will have trouble thinking clearly the next day. That goes for anyone, but for those with ADHD, it is all the more noticeable.

Dr. Colon also equates how we use our brain to the functioning of an automobile. As we build up waste products in our body and mind, those waste products impede our ability to function. Our metabolism takes in calories and expels waste products, just as a car takes in gas and expels exhaust, he notes. These physical and mental waste products build up throughout the day and, ideally, they're expelled during restful, restorative sleep. But if you don't get enough sleep, you're not fully cleansing your body of those waste products.

David D. Nowell, PhD, is a clinical neuropsychologist based in Massachusetts. He works with many adults who have ADHD. When he's not seeing patients in Massachusetts, he is traveling around the country giving workshops and trainings on ADHD. David has what he calls his "Big 5" when he works with adults with ADHD, and at the top of that list are sleep habits.

He suggests no screens in the bedroom, meaning no television, no tablets, and no smartphones. He says you should be in bed before midnight and up before 7 a.m. Once you get that habit down, he feels that you are then free to monitor your sleep habits and adjust them accordingly. But if you're staying up until 3 a.m. most nights, your sleep habits are not going to help you manage your ADHD during the rest of the day when you actually need to be awake and productive.

Dr. Nowell also suggests taking a hard look at caffeine intake. Find out how much you need during the day, as well as when you need to cut off caffeine for the day.

Dr. Colon says that your bedroom should be for sleeping. "One of the things I emphasize is making sure your room is a place for sleep." He also recommends anywhere from a half hour to an hour before bedtime to try to disengage from exciting behaviors. Once again: no social media, Candy Crush, work emails, or fast-paced TV shows.

If you do have a television in the bedroom, he has a little advice. He says that you should try to stay away from programming that is very stimulating, such as football. It will just keep you ramped up, and you'll have a tougher time slowing your brain down for sleep.

"When I was a kid, I actually did have a TV in my room," says Dr. Colon. "I used to love maps. It was a calming, soothing thing for me when I would look at a globe and think about different places and different cultures. When I was in high school and I would go to sleep, I would put on the Weather Channel because there were always maps, and I would just drift off to sleep. I didn't realize I was doing it because of that, but it just worked for me."

He has written a wonderful book called *The Sleep Diet: A Novel Approach to Insomnia*. The book focuses on how you can change your habits to achieve a good night's sleep.

As you might imagine, exercise and a good night's sleep go hand in hand. "As you exercise more, you need to repair and heal. You heal in your sleep," Dr. Colon says. He adds that those who exercise on a regular basis during the day have been shown to have shorter sleep latency, meaning it takes them less time to fall asleep. Regular exercisers also have deeper and more restorative sleep.

The other way to work toward a better night's sleep is to practice relaxation, and that leads to us being able to more quickly and efficiently calm down our racing mind. There was a time when meditation was something only New Age folks practiced, or so it seemed. But over the years, meditation has become much more widely accepted as an extremely effective technique in bringing calm and stability to our "monkey mind."

Whether you call it mindfulness or meditation, developing the habit of calming your mind and body has more benefits than we could list in this book.

"Mindfulness techniques are [very important] in helping with sleep but also helping with focused attention," says Dr. Colon. While he was a young man going through medical school and his residency, mindfulness techniques were key to his ability to stay focused. So while practicing some type of mindfulness technique is a great way to calm the mind, it also has clear benefits in helping you stay focused during other parts of the day, and it can certainly help you fall asleep as well.

Breath work is a crucial component of meditation. "Breath work is very important and, just as you have a heart rate, you also have a brain rate, and your brain rate is your level of alertness. If you're agitated or anxious, your heart races, and guess what? Your mind races, too—and it doesn't slow down." This, according to Dr. Colon, can cause difficulty in getting to sleep. And I think we have all experienced this at one time or another—maybe more so for those of us with ADHD.

"The reason the breath work is important is that as you breathe in, your heart rate is variable, and when you breathe out, your heart rate slows, and if you're breathing out longer than you normally do and you're slowing down your respiratory rate, you're calming down your heart and you're also calming down your mind."

Master Chris Berlow is a sixth-degree black belt in Taekwondo and the owner of United Martial Arts Center in Briarcliff Manor, New York. Chris is also an avid practitioner of meditation and promotes it to all of his clients and students.

Chris agrees with studies indicating that meditation and mindfulness techniques slow down the brain waves. But meditation also works by helping us bring our thoughts to the surface. As those of us with ADHD know, we can have so many thoughts running around in our head that we end up getting nothing done because of all that clutter. Many of us are creative individuals by nature, so the ability to declutter our brains is vital to organizing our thoughts. Many of us with ADHD are known for spinning our wheels or procrastinating, and a cluttered mind may be one of the reasons that we get a reputation for failing to follow through on projects.

Chris feels that many times when we meditate, the solutions to challenges or issues we face are more likely to come to the surface. "Because your brain waves slow down, you get to relax," he points out. Chris also feels that in order for meditation to work, you have to be able to relax both your mind and your body. When you do this, your life energy can flow freely.

"When you have stress or worry or doubt and those thoughts are going a million miles per hour, it tenses everything up and then that thought energy is not able to flow freely and effortlessly," he notes. Chris brings up the example of when you are in the shower. Many of us get our best ideas in the shower. Nurturing feelings of being surrounded by warm water, coupled with being alone with your own thoughts, get your brain to relax.

So how do you begin a meditation practice if you've never done it before? Chris offers some advice and some simple techniques to get you started.

First of all, practice breathing. Breathing is the foundation for just about any meditation program. He suggests that you just start practicing breathing and learn to breathe properly. "Take deep, cleansing breaths. You don't have to be in meditation to do that. Those deep, cleansing breaths bring more oxygen into your system, oxygen to your brain, and that can calm your mind." He also suggests pushing out your lower stomach as you inhale, which may be counterintuitive.

Next try to meditate first thing in the morning. According to Chris, you should meditate before your mind spins out of control thinking about work, getting the kids off to school, and the many other things that may need to be done before you leave the house.

His third piece of advice is to start small. "Start at five minutes, and if your five minutes is comfortable, go to ten minutes and increase at five-minute intervals." To achieve the full effect and benefits of meditation, you need to get yourself up to at least half an hour, and if you can, increase to an hour. That seems like a lot for someone who has trouble calming her mind down to begin with, but keep trying and increase the time at your own pace.

Chris also suggests that you count your breaths. "By counting your breaths, it keeps you focused on your breathing. One, it helps you maintain a singular focus, and two, it keeps you breathing." Chris advises setting some goals for meditation. Start with ten breaths and then another ten. And keep adding as you feel comfortable. Those short-term goals will make implementing meditation in your life attainable, rather than daunting and uncomfortable.

Once you get really at ease with counting your breaths, Chris says you won't need to focus on your breathing; that's when you know you are starting to get the hang of this mindfulness thing and start to relax. He also says that's when the thoughts will really start to flow freely.

Now I know what you're thinking: I'm ADHD, and when the thoughts start flowing freely, I start to think about all kinds of things, and it's anything but relaxing. Chris advises you to start focusing on counting again to bring your focus back to your breath if you feel your anxiety level rising. You could also make a habit of doing a "mind dump" after your meditation, writing down all the thoughts you had during that session. You may have had some great ideas, so don't let them go into the abyss.

There are other forms of meditation besides those that Chris suggests, but what I like about Chris's way of mindfulness is that it's not complicated. Breathe in and breathe out. Count your breaths and relax your body. When you break it down like that, it seems fairly simple. It's up to you to discipline yourself to keep going.

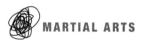 **MARTIAL ARTS**

Chris feels that those with ADHD are especially well-equipped to use their ability to hyperfocus to their advantage in the martial arts. "The need to be able to control your mind and body, to execute in a certain direction, I think feeds all the elements that an ADHD individual needs. There is constant stimulation, but it's stimulation in a productive way."

Practicing martial arts provides many benefits, and if you go to a school like the one Chris owns, you start your class with meditation and end the class with meditation. Each meditation session isn't an hour long, but rather a short session to get you relaxed for the class.

The physical activity will get that rush of dopamine flowing, of course. And there is that stimulation of the mind and body working as one for a specific objective. And martial arts is exciting and thrilling. Is it exhausting at times? Yes, but that will only help you sleep better. That said, Chris is adamant that you need to find the right martial arts school.

"I believe, as a martial arts instructor, that everyone has different personalities—there is no kid or adult who's the same. I've also learned that adults are just older kids. Every personality is going to be different, and what a good instructor needs to do is to find out what the student's personality is and what teaching tools are going to work with that individual. So if there's a student who's easily distracted with ADHD, I'm not going to give him five things in a row. I would give him one single focus and have him practice that."

Martial arts also provides a level of accountability. Some in the ADHD community do not like the term "accountability," but some of us need that in our lives. "The instructor at a good school is constantly and consistently holding the students accountable, especially as they advance," says Chris. As you learn more techniques and rise up in levels or rank, the expectations become even greater. And that helps you train to be more accountable for things you commit to.

If none of the many forms of martial arts is for you, consider other physical activities that might provide similar benefits: Yoga, group exercise classes, racquetball and tennis, or other pursuits can provide physical and mental exercise, accountability, and a reason to feel proud of yourself. You just have to find what suits you best.

But the research is clear. Exercise will help you manage and thrive with ADHD. It's up to you as to which kind of exercise you choose. Off to the gym!

CHAPTER SIX

the science of getting
nothing done

I was born in 1966, and that was a time when the medical profession did not have a name for what kids like me where going through. Not only that, they had no idea what we were experiencing in our minds. We were just hyperactive or problem kids. We didn't know how to behave, and I'll bet, in many cases, the parents were blamed for being bad parents. That was the doctors' simple answer for what is now understood to be a complicated mind-set.

And I think, to this day, there is still ignorance among those who do not have an ADHD child. They see the hyperactivity or worse out in public, and they immediately think to themselves that the parents are not disciplining their children and just letting them run wild. While that is certainly true in some cases, it's the first thing that comes to mind when we see kids acting out or misbehaving.

Many of us who fell into this category as children also sucked at school, and many I spoke with even got kicked out of school on numerous occasions. I remember sitting out in the hallway on many occasions in elementary school when I was asked to leave the classroom for being disruptive. And I remember the janitor walking by and sitting with me, asking me why I was sitting out in the hallway. It was a long time ago, but I'm guessing I probably didn't have a very good answer.

We were hyper, distracted, bored, and jittery all at the same time, and we ended up getting nothing accomplished unless we were threatened with discipline. And even in those times, many of us got little done that we were asked to do. And then we started to grow up and demands on our productivity got more intense. Schoolwork got more difficult and our attention to these important tasks waned even more.

Those with ADHD get a reputation for a whole host of traits, including being late, delivering tasks and projects late, or simply not doing them at all. We also have been known to procrastinate. We say we are going to do something, and time goes by and that something never gets done. Or, it gets done at the absolute last minute. And that leads to mistakes and a ton of unnecessary stress.

Wasting time and getting nothing done is not solely a trait of those with ADHD. We all do it at one time or another—so just because you can't get out of your own way doesn't mean you are ADHD. That being said, it's one of the major issues that adults with ADHD deal with.

Many people with ADHD are accused of laziness, but that is just the outward manifestation of a mind that, according to some experts, lacks the dopamine necessary to function correctly. That, plus what may be a self-defeating mind-set, gets in the way of productivity.

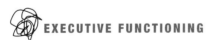 EXECUTIVE FUNCTIONING

Let's discuss "executive functioning." You may have heard this term, and you may have been diagnosed with what is called "executive function disorder." In short, executive functions help human beings plan and organize all their tasks.

We all engage in executive functions, whether we have ADHD or not. It's pretty much how the brain operates. Executive function is your brain's store manager. When you have good executive functioning, it is like your brain has a well-organized manager, his shirt is tucked in, he's wearing a nice tie, and his hair is neatly combed. The store (your brain) opens on time, and the staff knows what they are supposed to do. When you have problems with executive functioning, your manager is disorganized; he has a dirty, untucked shirt on, and his store is probably a mess. He has trouble getting to work on time and has issues with planning and delegation.

There is some confusion when it comes to executive functions and ADHD. Some people have been diagnosed with ADHD but not with executive function disorder. The reverse is true as well. And some in the medical field would argue that anyone with ADHD has some degree of difficulty with executive functions. But you can have issues with executive function and not be hyperactive. Does that mean you are not truly ADHD? Let a doctor decide.

"Executive function," when used in the context of executive function disorder or deficit—and I have seen both descriptors used—is an "umbrella term," according to Dr. David Nowell. In essence, executive functioning separates higher-functioning adults from others. Those with issues regarding executive functioning have trouble managing their time, achieving goals, and controlling their impulses. They also tend to procrastinate and have difficulty with planning and analyzing certain tasks. So when I say "higher functioning," I mean the ability to get stuff done. You may have a higher-functioning brain when it comes to creativity, as many with ADHD do, but when it comes to executive functions, we are talking about executable skills.

If you do have ADHD, you probably have at least some issues with executive function. Maybe not all of the above, but you most likely exhibit some of the characteristics. A proper diagnosis takes into account many factors and traits, not just being hyper and late for meetings.

Dr. Nowell creates a scenario for us that appears to enable someone with ADHD to thrive without many of the symptoms of ADHD or executive dysfunction:

You have a successful individual, around the age of forty-two. He fell into a business where he's doing very well, and the economy is working in his favor. In short, business is great, and he is thriving. His company is in a "zone," and his life is good. He has a great support system, both at work and at home. He married someone who has great executive functioning skills, and their home is tightly run. It's clean, organized, and things get done.

That same goes for this person's business. He has a great assistant as well as a support staff to ensure that the things he doesn't do well get done. This allows him to shine and focus on the things he does well—he spends time working *on* his business and not necessarily *in* his business. Maybe he is good at the overall vision of the business—say, its sales—and he can give a great presentation when needed. He is the face of the business, and everything else is running smoothly. He has the support needed to minimize the symptoms or traits that are associated with ADHD or executive dysfunction. We talked about the importance of a great foundation, and we will soon address in greater depth the concept of having a support system in place. This person has all that in place.

Then this person shows up in Dr. Nowell's office or the office of another ADHD professional. It may be because that support system fell apart, or the economy turned sour in this person's industry or business, and he lost the key components in his life that allowed him to shine.

The person in our story begins to eat poorly; his finances are catching up with him; he becomes incredibly disorganized; and, in general, his life starts to unravel, and his ADHD comes back to haunt him. And Dr. Nowell wonders why this person just showed up in the office of an ADHD professional at age forty-two. This person probably always had ADHD or ADHD symptoms and traits, but he had the perfect lifestyle and support system in place, and his ADHD never caused a negative impact on his adult life.

The point here is that this person may have always had ADHD or some type of executive functioning issues, and because of the chain of events in his life, he is now unable to get anything done. If he hadn't had a support system in place, these issues may have come to surface much earlier.

Dr. Nowell contends that, if he took time to look at this person's report cards from elementary school, he would most likely see those common comments we talk about with ADHD kids: "He can't sit still, needs to try harder, does not pay attention, does not complete assignments in the time allotted, not living up to his potential," and so on. Sound familiar? This person didn't just "come down" with ADHD or issues with executive dysfunction; they were always there, and he got things accomplished because he was surrounded by the proper supports and foundation he needed in his life.

"I think if you have all the right supports in line, you can really do well, and at that point you might say, what's the problem? On the other hand, adults who have ADHD often have an identifiable history of executive impairment," Dr. Nowell says. He talks about some of the common signs, such as a car being repossessed, a plummeting credit score, failed relationships, and vocational underachievement. To him, these would be huge red flags.

What is very common with those with ADHD is that we tend to do the things or tasks we enjoy and we don't do things that we find boring or, in some cases, challenging. That's why kids with ADHD do so poorly in school, because many of us were either bored, or we just didn't like what we were supposed to be doing. And we see this in hyperfocus: When we love what we are engaged in, nothing can break us away from it.

Many of us found something we love to do, have the proper support around us, and no one ever knew that we had a history of getting nothing done or executing poorly. We might have even forgotten about our own history. But we always have the type of brain that has some difficulty managing things inside our heads. We learn the skills and adapt to become productive and successful individuals. When these supports fail, we begin to fall into that familiar pattern of disorganization, inability to achieve goals, and lack of self-regulation.

Anyone with ADHD will have some issues with executive functioning. Our ability to implement strategies in our lives to help us deal with the type of brain that has been given to us is absolutely critical in not being labeled that person who never gets anything done, turns in work late, and procrastinates until it is painful.

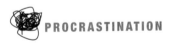 **PROCRASTINATION**

This might actually be one of the most talked-about traits of those with ADHD. And I've waited way too long to get to this part of the book. Get it?

After speaking with a few people about procrastination, I believe that it may be one of the most misunderstood traits of those with ADHD. At the same time, it's one of the simpler things to explain.

Procrastination is often viewed as laziness. And that may just be the case for some people, whether or not they have ADHD. Who doesn't want to sit on the sofa all day Sunday, watching football and eating ribs? Yeah, you need to cut the grass and clean out the garage, but that can wait, right? There are clear reasons that humans procrastinate. But there is a definite difference between procrastinating, being lazy, and putting things off in order to do other things. Because those with ADHD are easily distracted, drift off during conversations, and miss some of the details on occasion, we have a tendency to put things off. Why? Jay Carter is an ADHD coach, based in Minnesota, and he believes that when there is a lack of clarity in a task or project, those with ADHD tend to put it off. I agree with Jay's assessment. I know that when a client asks me to do something and she has not given me enough information to do it properly, I generally push it aside. Could I call and ask for clarity? Yes, but many times we simply wait until later.

Interest level is also a big part of procrastination. "If it's something I'm interested in and care about, I'm going to find that easy to do," says Jay. He cites the example of those in sales. Many people in sales, regardless of the product or service they promote, love sales. They love the thrill of the hunt and making the sale. But when it comes to doing the paperwork or their expense report, many are less enthusiastic. These parts of the job are boring, not very engaging, and don't make them feel good, so they put those off.

Tasks only get bigger and more stressful as time goes on. And as we approach a hard deadline, we are more apt to make a mistake or rush through what needs to be done. Rushing diminishes quality, and our work may appear inadequate and not up to standards set for us. Procrastination only causes stress, and it needs to be dealt with in order for us to manage and thrive with ADHD. We all put things off, but if that is part of the way we operate, it's a problem in the real world.

Timothy A. Pychyl, PhD, is a professor at Carleton University, Ottawa, in the Department of Psychology, who focuses his research on procrastination. He has written the book *Solving the*

Procrastination Puzzle and produces the *I Procrastinate* podcast. Dr. Pychyl believes that, in the case of those with ADHD, we might want to cut ourselves a little slack: "There are a lot of reasons for delay, and I think you can end up delaying things without it having the same sort of self-regulatory failure." He says it may not be fair to classify everything as procrastination when you take into consideration all the other things we deal with, such as attention, distraction, or organization. And he doesn't feel that it is fair, given all the other challenges that ADHD people face.

"Too many people use procrastination to cover all sorts of delay," Dr. Pychyl says. He adds that anyone can procrastinate, including those with ADHD, but we need to take into account that we might be experiencing other forms of delay and that certain delays can be a natural outcome of having ADHD. As we just discussed, Jay Carter feels that we procrastinate because of lack of clarity. Is that procrastination? We did deliberately delay the project in Jay's example because we were unclear about the specifics.

So, in Dr. Pychyl's words, what is procrastination? "Procrastination is a voluntary delay of an intended action despite being aware that you are going to be worse off because of this delay. It's important to understand that it's voluntary in the sense that if you're being forced to delay by circumstances or by other things then it's not procrastination, you're not culpable in that sense." You're voluntarily delaying it, nothing is preventing you from doing it, you've simply intended to do something and didn't. "All procrastination is delay but not all delay is procrastination."

He goes on to say that there are clearly other forms of delay, but procrastination is a negative form of delay, and it is self-defeating.

He thinks it's important for people who are challenged by various issues to take into account whether they want to call getting nothing done or procrastinating a moral failure. He feels that beating yourself up for endless procrastination demonstrates a lack of self-compassion and that consideration of your own ongoing issues is a key in overcoming procrastination.

So what drives procrastination? In other words, is there a science behind this trait? Dr. Pychyl explains that it is a self-regulation failure, like other self-regulation failures, including overeating and spending too much and gambling. "We have a desire to act in a certain way because we know not to is going to cost us, but we become our own worst enemy anyway."

Dr. Pychyl says that what we think of as a time management issue isn't that at all. "Procrastination is not a time management issue; it's an emotion-focused coping strategy. So really the self-regulation failure comes from in part an emotion regulation failure. We have the mistaken belief that we're going to feel better if we put something off, so that's our coping strategy—the delay to make ourselves feel better to avoid the negative emotions associated with a task."

Dr. Pychyl says the research shows that this is a misregulation not an underregulation: "We're not underregulating in the sense that we just put our minds to a particular task more. We have a mistaken belief that putting this off is actually going to make us feel better. But the fact remains that in the end, it makes us feel worse for putting it off. Short-term gain leads to long-term pain.

"It's clear to everyone that procrastination is a thief of time. Most of the time, our performance suffers." Procrastination is never helpful, and many times it is harmful to our productivity, and more, it can even end up becoming a health issue. "We feel very bad about ourselves, and oftentimes, our health will suffer," he says. In various research, heart disease and hypertension were found to be related to procrastination. He says that the shame and the guilt associated with procrastination can cause this unnecessary stress as well as the maladaptive coping mechanisms that occur as a result.

"Procrastination is a negative form of delay, and there is no upside to it," Dr. Pychyl points out. People want to believe that terms like "active procrastination" are a good thing, but he believes that is nothing but a misguided notion. The thought that active self-regulation failure is a good thing is somewhat erroneous. You don't choose to actively self-regulate failure. "Procrastination only has a downside, because it is a negative form of coping."

You and I can delay things for other reasons, such as purposeful delay, strategic delay, or delays that are inevitable because of other commitments, and we have delays due to mental health issues, such as depression. But we can't beat ourselves up for procrastinating, because other factors may impede our ability to get a task completed as well.

If we do procrastinate simply because it feels better to sit on the couch all day, we need to find ways to stop it and gain control of it so we can go on living our lives without constantly being behind on projects, tasks, and even more.

As you might imagine, impulsive behavior, another familiar trait of those with ADHD, may be closely linked to procrastination. "We see impulsivity as a big risk factor in procrastination because you can't protect one intention from another. So if you have a personality or a trait of being highly impulsive, then you're more likely to procrastinate," says Dr. Pychyl.

Low conscientiousness is another trait that has significant associations with procrastination. If you are low in conscientiousness, you are more likely to procrastinate as well. As Dr. Pychyl reports, "There is no doubt that impulsivity and lack of other self-regulatory skills and executive functioning skills are correlated with procrastination."

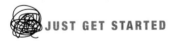 **JUST GET STARTED**

When I'm having trouble beginning a task, everyone tells me to just get started. Just do it. *What are you waiting for? Why isn't this done*

yet? But, according to Dr. Pychyl, it might be as simple as just getting started. And right about now you're saying, "Yeah, easy for you to say!"

"Most of us believe or have this mistaken belief that we have to be in the mood or feel like it," says Dr. Pychyl. He uses the example of asking your kids to do chores around the house. And, of course, the kid says he doesn't feel like doing those chores. Your response? As you might have said countless times before, "I didn't ask you if you felt like doing chores. It's time to do these things!"

He says that it's somewhat mythical to think that you have to be in the right frame of mind to get things done, because rarely are you in that "perfect state" to accomplish certain tasks. Now this might seem like it contradicts some of the advice you get as an ADHD adult—that is, to do the things you like to do and delegate the rest. But maybe not. If you are in a position in which you can't have someone else do some of the tasks you hate to do, guess what? You'll have to do them. You can't always delegate.

Dr. Pychyl suggests that a key element in just getting started on a task is to take your initial misgivings about how the task makes you feel out of the equation. No one loves doing the dishes or the laundry. But those things need to get done. So take the emotion out of it, or you'll have no clean dishes or clothing.

Just getting started sounds hard, but research has shown that it is one of the major factors in reducing procrastination. And once you start the task, you do start to get into the groove, and, in many cases, you make some decent progress and realize it's not that bad. It might even make you feel better. "The difference between a motivated person and an unmotivated person is what they are doing. And we've known from research that a little bit of progress in our goals improves our well-being," Dr. Pychyl explains.

Dr. David Nowell promotes the concept of "always be starting." Just employ the concept or mind-set that you should "always be starting" something—with, of course, the intention of completing whatever it is you're starting. We all know that those of us with ADHD love to start things and then never finish them. So many of us have a pile of projects on our desk that we want to get moving on, but we just don't seem to finish half of them. That being said, get into the mind-set of always trying to get started on those tasks. For those who maybe run a business and just have difficulty getting various tasks done, Dr. Nowell has a unique solution. He had the idea that he has seen others employ successfully. You can use video chats, such as Skype, to try what he calls the "body double" technique of getting things done. Have a set time you choose with a colleague to have that Skype support. She sits there in the background, and you both work hard to get those tasks done, supporting each other along the way. Establish a set time each week when you plan to complete those tasks you might otherwise procrastinate on. Working together, you can keep each other accountable and help each other through those important tasks.

On a behavioral level, just getting started is the foundation for getting things done. But, as Dr. Pychyl explains, it's not the only thing. There are also the cognitive aspects, as well as the emotional reasons, we procrastinate, and if you are a habitual procrastinator, you need to address that dynamic as well. He says that you need to understand the cognitive underpinnings of why you procrastinate and maybe even understand the irrational thinking behind your procrastination, along with the emotional feelings you get by doing or not doing something. Having the support of a therapist or even an ADHD coach can help you understand your own procrastination style and figure things out on a deeper level.

Life is full of ups and downs, regardless of who you are and what kind of personality you have. We might not like to do certain tasks, and we might not even like the job or career we are in. Most of us hate doing housework, and many don't care for food shopping.

But that's life. If you are rich, maybe you can hire someone to do your food shopping and cook your meals, but most of us are faced with tasks on a daily basis that just don't thrill us.

In this book you will find the advice that you should do what you love for a career or a job, if you can. And that is great advice. But it still doesn't guarantee total happiness in every minute of your day. "Even if we are interested in things, it doesn't mean we are going to wake up every day motivated," says Dr. Pychyl. Days on this earth are a roller-coaster ride, and the days we don't feel like doing anything don't mean we can wait for some divine intervention to get us off our ass. He says that all famous composers, actors, and other creative people practice their crafts daily. If you have to practice not procrastinating, then do it.

"Somewhere along the line we didn't get the message that grown-ups just do things, whether they want to or not," says ADHD coach Dana Rayburn. And we always think that we have to want to do what we need to do before we do it. Life doesn't work that way. As she says, "It's important to find things you are passionate about, but it's still not a cure-all."

lose the distractions and get in the zone

Those of us with ADHD are known for many traits, but one that sticks out is being distracted. However, distractions are not always bad. Sometimes they can lead to a great idea. But sometimes they can get you in trouble. While some ADHD traits, like the tendency to get distracted, get in the way of operating normally in a work environment, sometimes the same traits can give you an edge—that's what's so frustrating about ADHD. There were many times I was "wasting time" on social media and came across a great idea that we could bring to a client.

I use small distractions to remind myself of things I need to do. For example, I bring water from my home water cooler to the office in one-gallon jugs. I use these jugs to fill my coffee machine in the office, and then I bring them back home to fill them up. However, remembering to bring them home is not something I do all the time. So, I leave them right smack in the middle of the floor right in front of my office door all day. Their annoying presence in the middle of my floor sometimes gets me off track and certainly isn't organized in a traditional sense, but seeing them does remind me to take them home. Sometimes we need to actually trip over something to make it happen.

For many with ADHD, getting things done and accomplishing goals is one of the hardest things we deal with. In the case of procrastination, we learned that we often put things off simply because we don't feel like doing a particular task because it doesn't feel good at the moment. Others with ADHD put off tasks because they are generally disorganized to the point that nothing ever gets done and they lose track of the things they needed to be working on in the first place.

And then there are those of us who are just easily distracted. We have a tendency to be distracted by our own thoughts or things going on around us, but we are also more likely to let distractions enter our daily lives. These days, distractions are all around us, and ADHD adults are just a YouTube video away from getting thrown off track for hours.

When you are ADHD, discipline and willpower, along with self-regulation, are absolutely critical to getting anything done. Those who can muster the strength to stay off Facebook for more than an hour are far ahead of those who jump on social media every five minutes.

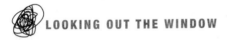 LOOKING OUT THE WINDOW

Dana Rayburn is an ADHD coach who lives in southern Oregon. She works with adults with ADHD, most of whom are small business owners and other successful individuals. Interestingly enough, she herself has ADHD, just like other ADHD coaches I have spoken with. Before becoming an ADHD coach, she was a professional organizer—not something you would think someone with ADHD would be good at. But she was good at it, and that led her to take the next step in her life by becoming an ADHD coach.

She grew up with ADHD, but she was not even diagnosed with it until she was in her thirties. She says she was an average student at best, but got better in college. As with many kids with ADHD, she tended to drift off when she was supposed to be doing something in school: "When I was in the fourth grade I had a teacher who sent us out independently, and we were supposed to write this gigantic report on Japan." It was a project that lasted a couple months and was supposed to be a showcase for the school's open house.

"My desk was next to the window, and I spent all those weeks when everyone was diligently writing their Japan report, staring out the window. So, for open house, my report was a cover page where I drew some cherry blossoms and then some blank pages. And I put that out there." And to her surprise, no one said a word about it, not even her parents. I asked Dana why she felt they didn't notice her unfinished project. She confessed that she didn't know the answer but she has often wondered the same thing. She believes that in the 1960s, not much was known about children that were inattentive due to ADHD. She believes that her parents felt she got bad grades because she was lazy and didn't do her work. She says a constant theme in her report cards was "Dana could be a good student if she would only try harder."

Another time, as an adult, after attending an ADHD conference, Dana was waiting for a connecting flight in the Salt Lake City airport. She had just left another inspiring conference, and as an ADHD coach, she had many friends in the business, so she was feeling great after spending time with everyone: "I was just on this euphoric high after the conference." Sitting in the airport, she was looking out the windows, watching the crews load and unload the planes. "I sat there thinking about how wonderful life was and what a gift life was and enjoying this moment and about an hour later I thought, 'Okay, I better mosey on over to my gate to catch my plane home.'" She went over to her gate, which was in another section of the airport and found out that the airline had been paging her for over twenty minutes. At that point her plane was pulling out of the gate, and she missed the flight. Because of this, she spent an additional ten hours in the airport.

Before she ended up being an ADHD coach, she worked in the corporate world in various positions. And just like the classic story of a person with ADHD, she took the ultimate risk at an earlier point in her life: quitting her job, traveling for a year, and moving to another state. Dana and her husband had great corporate jobs. Dana was a business systems analyst and a strategic planner for Hughes Aircraft Systems, later becoming a labor relations representative. Many with ADHD are risk-takers, and Dana was no different; she impulsively decided to quit a great job to see the country and the world.

After a year, Dana and her husband settled in Oregon, and she ultimately started her ADHD coaching practice, focusing on adults and business owners.

While Dana and I have no official coaching relationship, after speaking with her the first time about this book, she asked what my plan was to actually finish the book. In other words, "What would distract you from completing this task?"

"Well, that's a great question," I said at the time. Dana was keyed in on one of the traits of those with ADHD—distractions and leaving projects unfinished and deadlines unmet. It was a valid question, and it's true that I wouldn't have finished the book you're reading now if I hadn't had a plan and stuck to it.

Dana feels that the ADHD brain is constantly looking for something more exciting than what is currently going on. And those sounds, ideas, and thoughts ultimately cause distractions. According to her, this doesn't constitute failure; it's just the way the ADHD brain functions. She feels that one of the keys to being successful with ADHD is to get the internal chatter out of the way. And that involves a real-world approach, including brain care, mindfulness, and other techniques, as we noted in chapter 4 on building a foundation for living with ADHD.

Dana and others in her field feel that technology can be a distraction. On Dana's blog, she writes, "The Internet is like Alice in Wonderland falling down the rabbit hole. One link leads to the next."

Dana counsels her clients to conduct a short survey of the distractions around them. It's just like creating any other list of issues that need to be resolved. Once you know the actual distractions in your business life, you can then begin to tackle them one at a time. She suggests taking a few days to note what distracts you. You can then isolate what is causing these issues—you or an outside force—and then work toward changing the habits that guide you down the wrong path. For a business owner, distractions can be catastrophic and ultimately disastrous. By taking inventory of those distractions, you can be well on your way to eradicating those habits.

Many people who have created a thriving business or built a great career have found a way to minimize the distractions in their life so they can move their goals forward. While I might be a total multitasker when I clean the house, jumping from the dishes to vacuuming, this strategy doesn't work for most people when they're running a business. Some successful people may have figured out how to make it work, but I find that focusing your attention on whatever you are doing at the time is the best way to create the greatest accomplishments in business.

It's like one of the laws of branding a business. You can't be great at everything at the same time. Maybe you'll get things done, but not everything you do will be of the same quality as if you had shut out all the distractions and made one thing your priority. After all, we are really good at hyperfocusing, so why not use that to our advantage?

Dana suggests minimizing distractions in your daily life: "Be really honest with yourself on what the distractions are and then get rid of them." Dana also says that while our smartphones can provide some wonderful tools for managing ADHD, they can also be some of the most destructive devices for those with ADHD. With distractions it's important to learn how to buffer yourself against them as best you can.

It's also important, according to Dana, to manage how much stimulation you need to be productive. For many with ADHD, a completely quiet room with absolutely nothing going on is not the best environment for being productive. Again, it is totally an individual thing, but Dana suggests making sure that if you do need some type of stimulation going on where you work, you manage that properly. For me, it all depends. Some days I find myself putting the television on in the background in my office, and other days, I get halfway through the day before I realize it's not even on. The point is to understand what you need to be the most productive.

There are also internal and external distractions. Or to clarify this point, distractions, according to Dana, come from within ourselves, whereas interruptions come from other people. But, ultimately, interruptions become distractions—things that come into our conscious minds that shouldn't be there when we need to get things done. Maybe you need to shut your email program off or shut down social media. Shut off Skype or any other external interruptions that can end up being a distraction. "Put the squirrels in cages," says Dana. "We have to control what we are thinking internally in our brains, and we also have to control other people from coming in and bothering us." That may mean muting the phone or, if you work in an office, shutting the door when you really have to get things done—that is, if you have a door. If you work in a cubicle, getting things done can be challenging, because those with ADHD often take in everything going on in the office.

When you have a lot to do and you're feeling overwhelmed, take the time and space you need, if at all possible. If you need to work from home to catch up, sometimes that's the best option, if it's available to you. Working in an office as a manager can be a real challenge for those with ADHD. On the one hand, you do have a staff to do things for you and that you can delegate tasks and projects to. But you also have to manage that staff and have an awareness of what's going on with them.

ADHD coach Jay Carter suggests that you do everything you can to manage your environment. If you work for yourself, you can probably choose where you put your desk. But in an office setting, it might be a bit more challenging to get all the accommodations you need. Try to find the right location for your cubicle if you can, and set up your workstation so that you can function most effectively. That might include working on the side of the desk where you feel more comfortable and, if you need some extra light, adding a lamp to your desk. If you can escape to the conference room occasionally to get work done, try that. When you are at work, try to focus on those vital few tasks that are very important, and as many do, try to get those tasks done early in the morning. If you have to show up early when no one is in yet, you might opt to do that.

 THE MAYOR'S RIGHT-HAND MAN

Daniel Arrigg Koh has two degrees from Harvard University, worked for Mayor Thomas Menino in Boston, interned for Senator Edward Kennedy, and now serves as the chief of staff for the current mayor of Boston. And he's ADHD.

At fourteen years old, Daniel was not very worried about what a typical kid of that age was going through, such as getting a girlfriend, what high school would look like, and other age-appropriate concerns. He was concerned about how he could discipline himself to read a book. For his entire childhood he had trouble sitting still and reading. "It wasn't that I couldn't read," says Daniel, "it was that I could not get myself to sit down and read."

He often wondered whether he was just a procrastinator or if there was more to his inability to sit down and actually get through a book. When he was young, his parents always knew he was a bit hyperactive, but when Daniel was fourteen his mother, a doctor herself, read an article in the *New England Journal of Medicine* about ADHD and put the pieces together. Daniel exhibited many of the symptoms or characteristics that were specified in the article. His mother asked him if he wanted to get tested for ADHD, and he agreed.

"It was a struggle, because once you are diagnosed, you have a rationale or reason for why some of these things are happening to you," says Daniel. He points out that it's not as easy as just beginning to take medication and expecting the rest of your life to fall into place. "You have to compensate for the penchant your brain has to want to hop to the next thing." As a kid, this diagnosis required him to get up at the same time every day, as well as plan out his schedule methodically, and it also required having people around him who helped him stick to his routines and his schedule. His life after the diagnosis was very regimented, and to this day, David sticks to a regimen to keep on track.

 ## TWO DEGREES FROM HARVARD UNIVERSITY

Daniel earned two degrees from Harvard University. You don't think of that kid in your classroom who could not pay attention or had trouble reading going to Harvard, do you? Well, Daniel did, and it has served him well working in a field and a job that he loves. But it took him a little time to adjust to Harvard and find just the right combination of classroom studies and other activities to make it work for him.

Not until his junior year did he realize that he needed more out of Harvard than time spent just sitting in class and in study hall. He felt that being at Harvard, a school renowned for its academic rigor, compelled him to focus all his energy on his studies and sitting in the library all day. Expending the energy necessary to keep on task for such long periods left him exhausted and somewhat unfulfilled. So, in his junior year at Harvard, Daniel began taking up extracurricular activities and found that he could actually focus on his studies much better as a result of doing other activities. Even though it seems counterintuitive, having other channels for his energy, aside from the classroom and the library, relieved his fatigue and gave him the boost he needed to avoid burnout. He took up theater and a capella, and as a result, he found that he could focus more when it was time to work and study. Daniel's GPA went up 25 to 40 percent after joining these activities. He equates the feelings that he got after an a capella practice to how he feels after a workout. It was a creative outlet that he needed.

Daniel still needs to take part in other activities in his life. He is a marathoner and makes time to run every Saturday at the very least. "I found that with ADHD, one of the ways to live with the disorder is to establish a lot of habit in your life and establish clear goals, and knowing that I have a marathon looming forces me to go out and train." Every Saturday, just out of habit, Daniel goes out and does a thirteen-mile run. It helps him to clear his head but also prepares him for his next marathon. "If I don't do it, I go nuts, so it helps for me to establish that kind of regularity and helps discipline me to stay in shape."

"The severity of ADHD differs, and how to deal with it varies from person to person, so I don't think this is a cure-all, but it certainly was an important step for me that I realized I really should be pursuing these extracurricular activities, rather than fighting them and fighting my brain's penchant for wanting to do other things," Daniel says. These activities also allowed him to get to know other people he would not have had the opportunity to meet if he'd spent his college years sitting in the library studying all the time.

Daniel ultimately left Harvard University with an MBA, which led him to where he is today, working for the mayor of Boston.

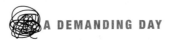 ## A DEMANDING DAY

Being in such a high-profile and demanding position requires Daniel to be regimented in his life. He gets up at the same time every morning, has a call with the mayor at 6:30 a.m., and eats the same thing every morning. At 8:30 a.m. he has a standing meeting with all the senior staff to go over the day's activities and make sure everyone is on the same page. Throughout the day, he has various meetings with the mayor, staff, and constituents. And, as a rule, none of his meetings last more than twenty minutes, because he believes that we have a tendency to want to discuss other things and get off track if a meeting doesn't have a predetermined time limit.

He leaves the office around 7 p.m., and then after dinner, at around 10:30 p.m., he has another call with the mayor to summarize the events of the day and make plans for the next one: a long but satisfying day.

Daniel feels that there are two parts of his job that would help someone with ADHD thrive. He has set up a structure in the office, and despite no day being the same—as you can imagine in the mayor's office of a major city—he has routines in place that enable him to serve the mayor well and lead his staff.

While not all of us with ADHD are good at multitasking, Daniel feels that it is a strength for him. Despite all the structure in place, he still works in the mayor's office of a huge city, and multitasking is a necessity. He cannot dwell on any one thing for too long, and he has to be able to work quickly and act accordingly most times. "This job, more than really any other, allows me to exercise some skills and a part of my brain that is my strength and allows me to be as effective as I think I can be," he explains.

"I need regularity, and I need structure in that way." Daniel feels that he has an advantage over others without ADHD because he has had to exercise that discipline. He feels that many without ADHD don't have the motivation to discipline themselves as he has in his life. He says that many times, those without ADHD can focus on tasks without being conscious of any particular difficulty, whereas he had to force himself to learn *how* to focus and even overcompensate by making meticulous task lists and strictly sticking to a schedule. These are skills he feels are important for someone to be successful in life, whether you have ADHD or not. ADHD simply gave him the motivation to cultivate and practice them.

Daniel started his foray into public service at an early age, working with local authorities to identify stores that were selling tobacco to minors. He was the kid who would go into the store and try to buy cigarettes. This was just the start of a career that has taken him to a job at the center of one of the busiest cities in the country. And he loves it. "I'm in a position now where if someone needs help in the city of Boston, I'm in a position to help them, and that's an incredibly humbling feeling, but it's also an incredibly exciting feeling."

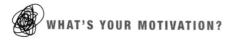 **WHAT'S YOUR MOTIVATION?**

"When you have ADHD, you have a certain humility because you know that your brain might not work like that of the average person." Daniel goes on to say that many with ADHD feel they have something to prove or overcome, and he believes that's an incredible motivator. "When I was a student in grammar school, I literally had teachers who wrote me off and said I never listened, that I was a lost cause, and all that stuff. That still sticks with me. Every time someone says I can't do something, I almost thrive off that because I heard that for a lot of my life, even when people didn't know I had this disorder; they just thought I was a kid who didn't listen, was distracted, and didn't care, and what I'm trying to do every day is to prove that kids with ADHD actually do care. They just have obstacles they need to overcome, just like everyone else."

He continues, "I think people with ADHD have to have a mentor or the mentality that just because they have the condition doesn't mean it's an excuse for achieving less in life. My parents right off the bat said we are not going to hold you to a lower standard just because you have ADHD. I think that the people with ADHD who say, 'Okay, I have this condition, how do I turn it into a strength and use that attitude?' are the ones who are really successful." Daniel feels that the proactive nature of people with ADHD is what makes them successful. "You live in a world where very few people feel bad for you, and you need to know that so you need to go out and find ways to make it a strength."

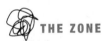 **THE ZONE**

Peter Shankman is a well-known entrepreneur and television commentator. You may have seen him talking on any number of cable network news shows about the latest company or celebrity facing various crises, or perhaps about what it takes to build a great brand, whether corporate or personal. He now describes himself as a "customer service futurist," helping organizations create loyal customers by having other customers share their stories. It's a little more involved than that, as you might imagine, but, in short, Peter teaches organizations how to create raving fans that sing their praises. He feels that the future of customer service lies less in price or service, than in the quality of the actual experience a customer has with an organization or brand.

Peter is probably best known for founding the very popular Help a Reporter Out (HARO) service, which connects reporters and journalists looking for resources to help them with stories. He also founded ShankMinds, which is a business mastermind program that has conducted entrepreneurial sessions in more than twenty-five cities. Additionally, Peter founded the podcast *Faster Than Normal*, which focuses on the strengths of having ADHD.

He started his career owning and running a very success-ful marketing and PR firm in New York City called the Geek Factory. Being well-known for creating PR stunts, he went on to write his first book about creating events or scenarios that would garner incredible amounts of press coverage and awareness in general for brands. For Peter, being creative and thinking unlike others in the PR world was totally in his wheelhouse. He has authored three books and knows how to get in the zone to get his books done.

It may have been his ADHD working overtime that came up with several off-the-wall ideas that brought incredible results for his clients: From a yarn bus traveling around the city for a knitting store, a 100-person skydiving event to promote his own company, to a web campaign that almost literally shut down the Internet, Peter has used some of the major features of his ADHD to his advantage. "What sane person would come up with a yarn mobile?" Peter confidently says. He also feels that this type of thinking gave him a clear advantage over other more corporate-style PR firms.

Peter is not shy about his ADHD—in fact, he embraces it. "I think it's a superpower, and it's really beneficial for me to have it," says Peter. "You want to have an incredibly fast car, as long as you understand and know how to drive it." And that's how Peter talks about his ADHD. To Peter, having ADHD and not knowing how to manage it or drive it can be a disaster, much like a fast car. "I think we are unique because we have tremendous brainpower, as long as we are able to correctly harness it."

One of the traits of an ADHD adult is risk taking. This may not extend to the extent of jumping out of a plane without a parachute, but in many instances, adults with ADHD are more likely to take a calculated risk in business and in life. And speaking of planes, in Peter's case, he is an avid skydiver and credits much of his creativity to the feeling he gets after a jump. "I think we are risk-takers because we see the beauty in things and we see the ability to create great things and to do new things to push the human race forward, but that doesn't come without risk. I also feel that there is a side of us that actually enjoys the risk." Peter feels that risk raises the dopamine levels in our brain and feeds that need to be creative and feel good. But he also feels that most ADHD adults take very *calculated* risks, and many of us do take the initiative to understand that the rewards must outweigh the risk before pulling the trigger on that next great idea.

For Peter, the Internet is a distraction, as it is for many of us. "When I get on airplanes where there is no Internet, I tend to work a lot better." Peter has written three books now, and each time, to avoid distractions, he gets on a plane and writes his book. Aside from a cabin in the woods, a plane 36,000 feet in the air is about as remote as you can get.

His last book about customer service was written as he flew from New York to California and back again; he wrote the entire book on the plane. In order to get his book done, Peter shut out pretty much everything, including the Internet. "For me, it's really about finding a place where I'm not distracted, where I'm able to get into a zone and really get to work." When Peter is in his zone, he essentially shuts out the world. He shuts out emails and stops checking his phone and anything else that might throw him off track. "The goal is to stay in that zone."

"I focus on writing after a workout. I'll work out and sit down and immediately get on the computer and start writing. My endorphins are such that I'm able to do tremendous amounts of work in a short period of time because of the way my brain is."

Peter also embraces a simple concept in eliminating choice. "I do my best in my day-to-day life when there are fewer options and distractions that can lead me down a wrong path. The ability to eliminate certain opportunities for me is very beneficial. If I eliminate choice, it eliminates risk, and it just seems to work better for me. I do know that I am very all-or-nothing, and a lot of ADHD people are, so, for me, it works in my favor."

Peter discusses what he calls "danger zones," and one big one for anyone with ADHD is a lack of deadlines. "When I don't write things down, that's a danger zone; if I'm not documenting things and I don't have a time when something's due, that's a problem. Deadlines are very key for me, so when someone says, 'Whenever you have it,' it never gets done."

Under the category of doing what you love, Peter now travels the world giving keynote speeches about customer service, marketing, PR, and other topics that he feels passionate about. He's one of the hottest speakers on the circuit when it comes to marketing. And it's the one place where he never gets distracted. And it may just come right back to being in the zone. For Peter, being in the zone is definitely being onstage. As he says, "Being onstage is the best thing in the world, that's where my life is 100 percent going and having a blast and everything's working perfectly. When I'm onstage the endorphins are flowing, life is running, and I'm just in a perfect world being onstage twenty-four hours a day."

EARLY TO BED, EARLY TO RISE

Peter is up by 4:00 a.m. every morning. "Doing that allows me to do a bunch of things. First, it allows me to go to the gym, and it lets me get work done because no one is up until 6:00 a.m. He gets into the office before 7:00 a.m., and that way he doesn't get bothered by other distractions. Peter says that getting in very early actually gives him a sense of control over his day. "If I come in the office at 9:00 a.m. and I have a hundred things I have to do and people are emailing and calling me, then my day is shot. That super-early rise is hands down the best thing.

Peter was not always an early riser, and like many of us, he needed to get in the habit of getting up very early. But he says that the benefits of going to bed early and getting up early far outweigh staying up all hours of the night. "I can count on one hand the number of good things that actually happened by me going to bed at 2:00 a.m. But on the flip side, I can count on multiple hands the things I missed out on. For me, I just realized that there is a big benefit to what I'm getting out of mornings, and my success comes from that; and the younger me always wanted to be successful, so that's what you do."

Peter trained himself to get up early by first quitting drinking. While he would ordinarily have a drink at night, he went to bed early instead. "I try to recall what it feels like when I do get up early and I'm satisfied, as opposed to when I wake up super-early and I'm exhausted. I try to play the tape forward and see what the benefits or negatives are of going to bed early or staying up."

Peter also enjoys getting up early because no one else is up. "It really is my time." His wife and child are still in bed, and it's his time to relax and start his busy day.

At night, Peter is usually in bed by 9:00 p.m. "What I've learned is there is nothing wrong with that." Some might tell him that he is missing out on certain things, but he doesn't feel that way. He doesn't drink, so he's not out all night hitting the best parties or at clubs. "If there are dinners that are important, I go to them. Other than that, I really don't miss out on anything."

Peter sleeps in his gym clothes so when he gets up in the morning, he hits the gym without having to decide what to wear there. "Not thinking about what I have to wear in the morning is a game-changer because it's one less thing I have to think about."

While not an option for many of us, Peter tries to keep his meetings to one day a week. That allows him to get all those meetings in, stay in that meeting frame of mind, and leave the rest of the week for producing results.

In terms of keeping to your routines, Peter advises understanding the triggers that cause you to deviate from your routines and finding ways to eliminate them.

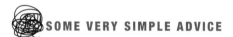 ## SOME VERY SIMPLE ADVICE

ADHD coach Jonathan Carroll has some very simple advice for those with ADHD who seem stuck: "You jump in headfirst and you just get it done," says Jonathan. You might not like hearing that, but even those with ADHD can muster the energy to clean the oven, which is what he was going to do right after our call. "I think that for things that you don't like to do, you've just got to do them." He also says that some things are interrelated, and if you don't do one thing, it can cause an entire process to fail.

Jonathan says that many with ADHD struggle to just get started on tasks. Cleaning the oven sucks, but it needs to get done so you don't burn your house down. And creating "to-do" lists is also important, but if you don't do what's on your list, what good is it? "I think that one of the challenges people with ADHD struggle with sometimes is that to-do lists are only as good as what they are written on. You can put off the items on your to-do lists, but as time goes on, more things get added to that list. And that can become overwhelming." He adds, "A lot of people with ADHD just keep putting things on their mental credit card."

ADHD coach Brendan Mahan notes that a good technique for those with ADHD is to begin a project with the end in mind. And while this is certainly not an earth-shattering insight, it is good advice for a person with ADHD because, in many cases, we do have the end in mind; we just don't pay much attention to the details that are needed to get something done. "Envision your end as clearly as possible, and then figure out how to build to that end by working backward, from it." If you don't think you can do an entire project for work in one session, break up the task or project into smaller pieces. We talk about the Pomodoro Technique™ in the next chapter, which is a great way to break things up and get the mental break you need to plow through a ton of work.

Also, keep in mind that ADHD does not automatically mean being lazy. Eric Tivers does a presentation where he describes a person lying on a beach and he describes that as lazy. "Lazy is the *choice* of inactivity," says Eric. Thinking about all the things that you need to do and not doing those things—that is not lazy, that is executive dysfunction. Eric goes on to say that motivation is not a character trait, it is a neurological feature. He explains that when we start thinking about motivation, we need to ask what we need to do to get the brain to do what we need it to do.

We mentioned the concept of the mind dump earlier, and Eric agrees that this is a great technique for understanding how to plow through certain projects and tasks. In short, get everything out of your mind and onto paper or some kind of technology. "Our ability to hold a number of pieces of information in our mind at any given time is very limited. Our brain is not good at storage of temporary information; it's good at problem solving." So what we want to do is get all those floating pieces of information on paper or in some type of software, such as Evernote or another organizational program. Eric says the goal is to see it all and then begin to work with it.

Eric starts by having his clients go through the lists and find those tasks that they feel will take between five and fifteen minutes. He has them separate those out, and then he asks if any of these tasks have been floating around for a long time. He says that giving yourself permission to take certain tasks off your list is okay. He has even had some of his clients create a "not now" list. This kind of separation is a good way of keeping that task or project somewhere, without the daily reminder that it's not getting done.

Eric then works with his clients to develop time horizons for projects and tasks. He asks what might be realistic over the next three months and even suggests that they go out a year if they feel they can. But he says that in most cases he works in quarterly periods with his clients. He then asks his clients to estimate how much time these tasks or projects will take, and they write that on the page right next to the project. The client will then use a stopwatch, start the task, and then record how long it takes for them to complete each one. Ultimately, they have a record of how long that particular task takes. Eric says you need to write this information down, because for most people with ADHD, trying to remember how long something takes is just a bad idea. Write it down, and have a record of it to refer back to it next time.

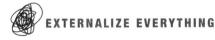 **EXTERNALIZE EVERYTHING**

I mentioned earlier that I put the water jugs right near my office door when they need to be filled so I pretty much trip over them. That's one way of externalizing what you need to get done. But another way is just to make sure that anything you need to get done comes out of your brain and is placed on something. Make sure you have a working written or typed to-do list. Create charts and cards that help your working memory, and use those to make up for your inability to remember things that are important. Use software, such as Evernote, to compile these important notes and tasks, or simply write them down on a legal pad. Whatever works for you. I have talked to several people who swear by technology and others, like me, who just use a good old-fashioned written to-do list. But whatever you do, make sure you do it.

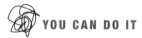 ## YOU CAN DO IT

For many of us with ADHD, our mind takes over, and when that happens, we have a hard time producing results. We think things might take longer than they actually do, and our mind tells us that these things are just too hard to get started on. We also misjudge the amount of time it will take to complete a certain task, and we either end up not completing it or we get it done late.

If you are going to be a successful business owner or find a career that you want to excel at or just get through college, you have to be able to get things done, plain and simple. In elementary school, if you don't get your work done, you get a bad grade. In the real world, if you don't get things done, you lose your job or you lose a client.

routines and time management

Let's face it, those of us with ADHD can watch the time fade away without even knowing it sometimes. Or, we can get going on something that wasn't in our schedule and absolutely lose track of time. We cannot get time back on this earth. There are only twenty-four hours in a day, and if we waste our time without a plan or a way to make sure we maximize our time, then all of sudden it's Friday and we realize we got nothing done, yet again. Hop on YouTube for a quick tutorial on how to shoot video for your business and all of a sudden you're watching videos of Caribbean beaches. Not that I've ever done that, I just know a guy who did.

As we've discussed, you have a basic understanding of how you work. So when it comes to managing your time, all the advice in the world won't stick with you unless you keep that basic understanding in mind. Many of the professionals we consulted for this book can tell you that you need to go to the gym in the morning, but if your office is sixty miles away from the nearest gym and you need to be in the office by 7 a.m., that routine probably won't work for you. Or maybe your energy level really peaks at a different time during the day. Maybe you like to go to the gym after dinner or on your lunch break. It's your choice as to how you manage your time. But starting your day off on the right track is critical, regardless of whether it starts on a treadmill or with a moment of meditation. And you need to develop a routine if you are going to thrive with ADHD.

When you wake up in the morning, what do you do? Have you ever written down your morning ritual, or the lack of one? Do you have any idea how long it takes you to get out of the house? And, if you have an early morning meeting somewhere other than your office, can you estimate how long it will take you to get up, get moving, and get there on time? Many with ADHD can't answer these questions. And many with ADHD just let time pass without having a say in how it's used.

"Routine is very important," says Jonathan Carroll, an ADHD coach based near Chicago. "You always have to act *as if.*" What he means is that if you just show up to your business without some type of purpose or strategy for managing your day, things can get out of control very quickly. He describes a hypothetical unemployed person. Instead of just sitting around the house all day, waiting for the phone to ring, he would tell this person to get up as she normally would if she were working, then eat, shower, get dressed, and go out and do something productive. "I think we have to have routines, almost to an obsessive-compulsive [extent]." Jonathan says that obviously we have to be adaptable, given the circumstances of life, but having no routine is not an option.

It's also important to have a place for the things you might need before you leave the house each day, such as your keys, briefcase, phone, and other essential items. If you don't have a place for them, you'll end up wasting time trying to locate them. Or, even worse, you might get all the way to the office before realizing you forgot something important, which causes a whole other level of stress.

Habits are good for those with ADHD as well—they just need to be good habits. Our goal is to work toward having more good habits than bad ones. "Those of us with ADHD tend to go on autopilot when we don't have autopilot in place yet," says Eric Tivers. "We need to be intentional with everything we're doing." That includes your routines for various parts of your day, as well as your overall scheduling. "As many of these processes as we can automate and systematize, the less we have to use our executive function," says Eric.

 ## FROM FLIPPING DESKS TO HIGH PRODUCER

Routines also help us get off on the right track, especially in the morning. For Greg McDaniel, they are absolutely critical in helping him be a high-producing real estate professional. Routines give us a solid footing for the day and set the tone for how we will attack our life for the next eighteen hours. That's just why Greg has a morning ritual as well as a plan of attack when he gets to his office.

It wasn't always that way for Greg. As with many kids with ADHD, his childhood was turbulent at times. Greg also has dyslexia, so in elementary school, he had challenges reading and writing, which was a huge source of frustration. He was taken to doctors, and at first they thought he had brain cancer, but after many tests, it was determined that he had ADHD and dyslexia.

He was transferred to a different school that specialized in helping children with learning disabilities. At the time, he thought it was an awful experience. His days were spent watching and listening to teachers phonetically spell and sound out words. "Looking back, it was a good thing, but going through it, I thought it was the dumbest thing ever." This led to behavior issues, including flipping desks over and other forms of acting out.

Greg finally came to the conclusion that he might be a little different, at least in the neurotypical sense, and began to take medication to help with his ADHD. The medication helped him get through school, but he admits to only doing the bare minimum he could get away with in grade school all the way through junior high and high school. He says he was at best a pretty good C student. He got an A– one semester, and he thought that was the best day of his life.

He finally went off to college but ended up turning that into one big party. For Greg, college consisted of nonstop drinking and eating fast food. Again, he wasn't being taught the way he needed to learn, so the result was more frustration, which resulted in his excessive lifestyle.

He says his schooling was disappointing, but his difficulties did teach him valuable lessons. After school, he ended up with a job in the real estate business, and in 2008, he lost almost everything. Many others in real estate lost quite a bit as well during that year, so he was not alone, but that certainly didn't make the experience any better. In the next few years, he clawed his way back to solvency. He used his likability to carve out a niche for himself: prospecting. In other words, he came to understand that he was very good at getting out there and generating business. Some people would blanch in horror at making thousands of cold calls, but Greg did it with intense focus, and he slowly built his business back up.

Today, aside from being very successful in the real estate market, Greg also produces a popular real estate podcast called *Real Estate Uncensored*. Greg is very engaging and covers a wide range of topics to help other real estate agents maximize their business. If you watch his videos on YouTube, you will see how personable he is, which is a gift.

In order to be a high-producing real estate agent and crank our regular podcasts and videos, he needs a regimented day to keep everything going and to stay motivated. Greg sets his alarm for 5:00 a.m. every day. Maybe hits the snooze button once, but that's it. He turns the light on and says to himself, "It's going to be an amazing day!" His feet hit the floor, and he says it again. "Today is going to be an amazing day!" He says that once his feet hit the ground, he is fully committed to making his day great. He throws some cold water on his face, feeds the cats, and he's out the door to the gym. After an hour-long workout, he's back to the house to get ready for his amazing day.

He has a thirty-minute drive to his office, so that allows him to listen to a podcast or a motivational book on the way to his office. Once he's in the office, he blocks out a minimum of one to three hours for prospecting and outbound calls. His calendar has everything on it, so there is no doubt about what he needs to be doing. As he says, "I live and die by my calendar."

Greg has to include that prospecting in his calendar every day, rather than just leaving it for when he feels like it, or for some future unscheduled moment. Prospecting is very important in his business, and it's more effective for him to have a certain time to do it. "I have to do my prospecting every day. Some form of it, I have to do because it's my lifeblood. If I don't prospect, I don't eat. I like to eat—lots—so I need to prospect a lot." Many people don't like prospecting or what we might call cold calling, but he says he's come to like it because he's good at it.

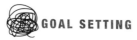 GOAL SETTING

Greg also has one other thing he focuses on every day, and that's his goals. He has a wonderful system that allows him to literally visualize his goals: He has a "dream book" and a "dream wall" in his office. He writes or types his two-year goals, then lays them out in the book. He includes financial, business and career, achievement, fun and recreation, health and fitness, relationships, as well as self-improvement and educational goals. He is constantly updating his goals to make sure they align with his values and vision for his life. The thing about goals, in Greg's mind, is that you need to state your goals in the present, such as "I am," "I have," and so on. He recommends that you don't say, "I will" or "I might." He feels that you need to be in the present mind-set for goals to be reached. "You need to be crystal clear on what you want." Greg believes that 95 percent of the time, when you write your goals down and review them on a daily basis, those goals get achieved.

Greg's desk also faces his dream wall. It's covered with things he wants and goals he needs to achieve, as well as inspirational material: the car he wants to buy, great quotes to keep him motivated throughout the day, and so much more. In short, Greg has the mind-set that when he states his goals, he's saying, "It's going to happen."

"You can literally create anything in your future and in your life; all you have to do is write it down, and then have fun looking at it and thinking about it and enjoying the positive feelings you get around it." Greg says that, among other things he's incorporated into his life, goal setting is by far the most effective way he manages his ADHD. "If you remind yourself about what you're working for and what you're doing it for and what you want and you really get excited about doing it, then you can take your ADHD and put it in the backseat, because you'll have a bigger reason and a bigger 'why' to get up and go do what you need to do. If you have a why, you will make it happen."

Of course, everyone is different, as we all know, but Greg says that the most important thing for those with ADHD is to have a why. He recommends finding your why and building your goals around it. That will help you build a path and hit the ground running. He says it's all right for your goals to change during the journey, too, since we all evolve and progress throughout our lives, but as long as you constantly have those goals in front of you, you'll have something to work for. Greg takes pleasure in working toward his goals every day, and he feels it has been vital to managing his ADHD and becoming successful and a positive thinker.

Greg says, "If I want certain things in my life, then I have to have a routine put in place. Nothing comes easily, and nothing comes for free, so if you want to have a good body, you have to go to the gym. If you want to have a strong mind, you have to read and learn. If you want to become wealthy and successful, you have to put the time and energy into it." He says his goals and his dream wall are very important parts of his routine because he reviews them regularly so he can keep heading right toward his goals. He says that if you don't have a routine, getting to your destination is nearly impossible.

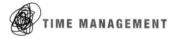 **TIME MANAGEMENT**

Many in the ADHD community say that we don't have a motivation problem. The real problem is time management. To carry this thought one step further, we sometimes don't even understand the consequences of poor time management until it's too late. Getting long-term projects done and off our desk may be even more challenging. Yes, many of us have the ability to hyperfocus but, by the same token, we are also pulled away from tasks by any number of outside variables.

To say there have been countless books on time management written over the years would be an understatement. Maybe you have read a few of them. Or maybe you meant to read them, but just were never able to carve out the time. Whatever the case may be, proper time management for those with ADHD is critical. One, because many of us just lose track of time, but also because managing our time forces us to investigate how long we'll need for the various tasks that we must do to effectively live our lives. I have learned over the last few years that in order for me to get certain mission-critical tasks done in my business, I have to manage my time. I use Outlook™ to block out my day, but whatever you do, find a way to schedule your life.

It may sound basic and second nature for those without ADHD, but Dr. David Nowell says that you have to schedule your day *in advance*. He says that if you leave large unstructured blocks of time in your calendar, it's difficult for you to assess whether you are on track to complete your tasks or projects. Dr. Nowell suggests that you consider blocking your entire day out, not just the time periods in which you plan to work. Put your projects in there, the gym, and even dinner, if you need to—the more specifically you outline how your day is going to go, the more realistically you can evaluate what time you have. He also says that when you get to the late afternoon and your willpower is beginning to wane, you can look at your calendar and see what you should be doing to keep yourself on task.

Dr. Nowell also suggests that after you have been doing this for a while, you should reassess your progress. Go back through your day, and ask yourself whether you completed the projects you were trying to finish. If you went off schedule or a task took longer than you thought it would, decide where you might have gotten off track. See if any patterns emerge. In my case, I noticed that I usually deviated from my schedule in the later afternoons. Because I saw a pattern of lack of focus happening late in the afternoon, I started going to the gym during that time because I wanted to stay productive.

Dr. Nowell says that you should analyze if you are allowing enough time for tasks, or see if you are scheduling too many things back to back, or you are scheduling tasks or appointments when you

are at the end of the day and your energy is running low. And analyze when you do certain tasks. If you are creative in the morning,
use that time wisely. In short, maximize each hour of your day to
do the things that match that time of day and the energy you have
to go along with it.

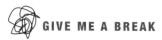 GIVE ME A BREAK

Another great way to maximize your time is to use the Pomodoro
Technique. If you are not familiar with this, let's run through it.
The Pomodoro Technique is very simple, but in my opinion, very
effective. It's loosely based off the kitchen timer that looks like a
tomato. Maybe you had one of these in your kitchen growing up.
In short, you set a timer for twenty-five minutes. Then you take a
five-minute break to clear your head. Then you set the timer again
for another twenty-five minutes, and then take another five-minute break. And so on. You can almost turn this into a game by
racking up many Pomodoros.

You can condition yourself to work in short little bursts with
that five-minute reward at the end. The break allows you time to
clear your head but also reminds you that you need to get back to
work for another twenty-five minutes. By knowing that you have
to work without interruption for a set period of time, it increases
your productivity and focus on a particular project or task. An entire
book and system has been developed around this technique, and
I encourage you to find the book and actually buy the Pomodoro
timer, if you're interested.

An alternative is the Pomodoro app, which you can download.
I have it on my phone, and it works great for me. The app allows me
to see how many sessions or Pomodoros I have managed to focus
through. In its truest form, in my opinion, the program represents
accountability to yourself. By following the Pomodoro plan, you are

telling yourself that you will be shutting out the world for twenty-five-minute bursts in order to get things done. You do it, and then you reward yourself at the end with a five-minute break. In essence, you condition your mind to focus on something for twenty-five minutes at a time. I love the Pomodoro app because you can use your phone to set its alarm to a short, relaxing New Age ring that says, "Hey, good job, take a break."

For your five-minute break, do something that relaxes your brain. Do something fun or something that you always have an urge to do, like hop on Facebook for a few minutes. Try not to do extra work, as that will continue to tap into the brain energy you will need for the next twenty-five-minute focus period.

The great thing about the Pomodoro Technique is if you have a very long task—say, writing a book—it's a great way to break it up. Dr. Nowell suggests that you try scheduling a fifteen-minute break for every three Pomodoros you achieve, or whatever you feel makes it easier to move forward. The great feature I found on the phone app is that you can tweak the timing of your work sessions as well as your breaks. So if you find that, to start with, you need to work for ten minutes and then take a break, you can set the timer to do that. You can also program the amount of time for the break. And of course, you can set the timer for more than twenty-five minutes if you feel it's appropriate. It's all up to you.

I personally came to love this technique very quickly. And maybe many of us have tried variations of this or looked at our clock to say we will work to a certain time, but having a physical timer that is programed to tell you when to work and when to take a break makes all the difference in the world. Still, you have to commit to not doing anything else while you work, and that means no social media, not even for a minute. Don't do it. Stay focused and maybe even try to compete with yourself to see how many sessions you can complete successfully. Look at that timer and say, great, I only have ten more minutes and then I can get up and take a break. And when that sound goes off again, sit back down and get to work.

You don't have to use the actual Pomodoro timer to make this work for you. There are other similar methods that you could use or come up with if you choose. The whole idea is to commit to working for a set period of time and then reward yourself with a break. The idea is to benefit from the relationship between work and reward.

Dr. Nowell suggests that even using a streaming music app like Pandora can create a similar environment, but make sure it's the free version, because it has advertisements. I know, you're saying, "Why?" Because you hate commercials. But they can actually help you be more productive in this case. When you listen to streaming radio, after a few songs, you will normally hear an advertisement. The idea is that you work when the music is on and you break during the commercials. Get up, stretch, see if you are still on task, and when the music comes back on, get back to work.

At this point, I don't have any set timing when it comes to working and taking breaks at the office. I know I'll need to get up and walk around after a period of time, but I rely on my intuition to understand when the time for a break has arrived. I use the Pomodoro Technique for longer or more intense projects when this less structured approach to work is no longer rigorous enough. It really has changed the way I get things done. One, because I like to achieve goals. With Pomodoro, they may be small goals, but completing the process successfully makes you feel good. The second reason this technique works for me is that it's a struggle for me not to continually check social media. Working in marketing and public relations and being responsible for several client social media platforms, it's easy for me to justify browsing Facebook for work reasons, but I often end up getting sucked into something else while I'm just keeping abreast of my newsfeed. I've found that knowing when I can and cannot do certain things like that is crucial for productivity.

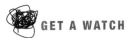

GET A WATCH

OK, another very simple yet important detail in managing your ADHD is getting a watch. But, you may be saying, I use my phone! Isn't that enough? Yes, it does tell you the time, but for many with ADHD, a *constant* reminder really makes the difference. And, of course, unless you have an Apple watch, your timepiece won't have Facebook, Twitter, games, music, and all the other fun and distracting things that populate your phone. A watch is usually just a watch. With a watch, it's a matter of turning your arm over, seeing what time it is, and going back to what you were doing. But look at your phone to see the time, and all of a sudden you're chatting with friends on Facebook and doing seven other things you shouldn't be doing.

Eric Tivers also says that you should have real clocks around you and timers to help you get things done. Eric points out that many with ADHD are "time-blind," so the more clocks and timers around you, the better.

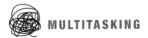

MULTITASKING

Multitasking was a big word back in the 1980s, and it most likely came into your vocabulary when we started to see the personal computer pop up in the workplace and at home. But for those who have ADHD, it was a thing before it was a thing, if you know what I mean.

Spencer Shulem is an app developer who created his first app at the age of thirteen. He goes against my suspicion that multitasking is a recipe for disaster for adults with ADHD. He feels that he can get quite a bit accomplished by multitasking—as long as he sets boundaries. I feel that focusing on one task at a time breeds quality results, even though it may take more time. For many of us, if we try to do too much at once, that can lead to mistakes. But then there are those who swear by it.

Spencer says that the hardest part about multitasking is that you could end up getting nothing done. If you don't do it right, multitasking can easily lead to starting twenty things and finishing zero. He says, "How I've made it work for me is really understanding what I need to get done and when I need to get it done. When I have those two parameters in place, I can start one hundred things and sure, it might take me a week to finish those one hundred things, but that's when I need to get it done. So I can just systematically go through what I need to get done." For those with ADHD, this can work. Your mind may be racing and says no, don't look at one thing—let's look at ten other things. If looking at those ten other things causes you to completely lose focus, multitasking isn't for you. But if you can let your brain run free and find a way to maintain enough focus to complete all those other things, perhaps multitasking is for you.

Spencer says he also has OCD, obsessive-compulsive disorder. As a child, he was diagnosed with OCD, alongside his ADHD. "With my OCD, I really need things to be really clean and really perfect. And that causes me to have to [eliminate] clutter. So when I have twenty things open, I really want it to be one thing. I want to open my desktop and have one task." He says that merging multitasking and what he calls his OCD does actually work for him. "I don't think I'm unique, and no one wants clutter," he explains.

As Spencer and I were doing a video chat for this book, he told me that he had two computers on his desk and had about fifty windows open. But at the same time, I did have his attention, and I wouldn't have known he had all this going on in the background if he hadn't told me. Spencer may have plenty of tasks in motion at any given time, but he sets boundaries and knows that in order for him to move on to the next five items on his to-do list, he has to finish the first five that are in progress.

Spencer does admit that you probably can't truly multitask in the sense of doing two difficult and ultimately different tasks at the same time. "But," he says, "to be able to work on a lot of things simultaneously has been incredible, but you have to set yourself those parameters." He also states that, yes, if you need to work on software design, then on programming, and then preparing for a venture capital meeting, then, yes, of course, each of those tasks do require your full attention. You can't successfully do them all at once. But in the office, sitting at his desk, expect to see him working on multiple smaller tasks that don't demand his full attention.

I asked Spencer whether, if he were told how to stop multitasking, he would take that advice, and he said flat out that he would refuse. He says that if you have to manage anything, such as a business or a division of a company, then you can't really avoid multitasking. I agree with that, based on my own experience, and to this day, there are times when I too have multiple windows open on my computer. I may be working on a particular project and then find a resource that I can use for something else. I might leave that website open on my computer for hours before I circle back and do anything with it. There's no way to completely eliminate multitasking from your life, so it's important to understand how to handle it, whether you have ADHD or not.

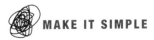 **MAKE IT SIMPLE**

My personal opinion is this: Make it simple. Make your schedule simple, and make your task and to-do lists simple. Have a simple routine at night and in the morning, and don't create an overwhelming set of things you need to do to get out the door. Part of time management when you have ADHD is setting things up in advance, knowing what your day is going to look like, and creating an environment where you can do whatever you need to get done. Make your lunch and the kids' lunches the night before. Cook a bunch of food on Sunday, and make those meals last a few days into the week so you don't have to cook every night. Lay your clothes out the night before, and have your keys, wallet, and briefcase ready and in the same place. These are just some of the tips that might help you put together a routine of your own.

Start the day off on the wrong foot—get up late, run around the house to get the kids on the bus, and forget everything you need for work—and good luck getting anything done all day. By developing a solid routine and working on your time management skills, you can get up on time, prepare your day in advance, and use those proven techniques for getting things done. At the end of the day, you'll be a happier person.

CHAPTER NINE

making ADHD work *for* you

I believe that ADHD is a gift. Yes, a ton of negatives come with it, and if we survive elementary school and beyond, including getting kicked out or sent to special education classes, we can do great things and come up with amazing ideas. There have been countless adults with ADHD who had a history of report cards that were dismal, to say the least. And those report cards didn't help our self-esteem, either.

Any of the following comments sound familiar? "Has difficulty completing class assignments in a timely manner. Needs to work on sitting still and focusing on class lessons. Needs to work on following directions. Has difficulty concentrating. Needs reminders to stay focused during the school day. He's great at art." Aside from the last one, these comments stay with us, and we need to realize that, in spite of that early criticism, we do have something to contribute. It just might have to be on our own terms.

Kicked out of school in the fifth grade, Spencer Shulem, whom we met in the last chapter, was one of those ADHD kids. He didn't have the academic struggle that other kids might have had, but he was a classic case of an ADHD child, jumping from one task to another and lacking in the interpersonal skills necessary to relate to the kids around him. He explains that he was in fourth grade doing ninth-grade math but had real issues with focus.

"Growing up I had some of the worst ADHD people had ever seen," says Spencer. "It was a genuine and real struggle for me as I was younger, and on top of that, there was that pressure of 'now you have a disability' and there's the pressure of being treated differently and doing things differently, and you can't really follow the same guidelines as everyone else is, breezing through in life. And that was hard because when you're a kid you don't really understand what a disability is and you're also told that you have a disability."

Spencer felt that he was forced into a group of kids with all kinds of disabilities, including very severe mental and developmental issues, and that hurt his morale. "It's not that there is anything wrong with having a disability. It's just that when you are a kid you don't understand it and you don't understand what that means and what it is."

Spencer did well academically, but his focus was the issue. "The teachers would really get frustrated with me to the point where they would just keep punishing me. And that would frustrate me." There were weeks during elementary school that he was sent out of the classroom every day. Oftentimes, he was just sent home. In fifth grade he was kicked out of school. It was a private school, so they had the authority to ask him to leave. He ended up homeschooled and then eventually got into a charter school.

Spencer was always interested in technology, and he feels it was definitely one of his strengths, even in school. At summer camp he remembers the teachers telling his parents that they had run out of things to teach him, so Spencer ended up setting up computers for the summer camp.

"I just really loved technology, and I was sent home because of it. I would have this disobedient attitude. When the teacher was doing something wrong on the computer, I would say, 'You are doing it wrong' or 'You need to be doing it differently.'" That led to Spencer developing a bit of an attitude: He reveled in the personal victory of telling someone in authority what to do after having a childhood of having others tell him what to do.

Spencer says that when he got to high school, things changed. He went from the charter school, where they were very aware of his ADHD—or, as they classified it at the time, his "disability"— to the high school, where they were not aware of it. At that point he chose to ignore his ADHD. It was one of the best decisions he ever made.

"No one saw me getting extra test time, no one saw me having a disability, I didn't take drugs anymore; I just kind of ignored me having ADHD, and I just started working as if I was a kid who just had a hard time focusing," he says.

About the same time, his parents got a divorce. Spencer says that his mother was always very focused on what she thought was his disability, but after the divorce, they did not communicate every day. "I think not having someone around who was persistent on me having something wrong really helped me get out of this box of saying, 'There is something wrong with you.' And I think when you're told you can't focus for more than fifteen minutes, you're not going to be able to get a good grade in this class, you're not going to be able to take that test, you need more test time—when you're told that, it's kind of like a scapegoat."

He goes on to say that, for him, getting away from people telling him that he wasn't good enough helped him to improve his self-esteem. He decided that his mind-set was not going to be that of a person with ADHD but more of an individual who had his own strengths and weaknesses.

And he carries that mind-set with him in his professional life. He doesn't use his ADHD as an excuse for not getting things accomplished. "When I have a bad or unfocused day, I take full responsibility for it. I say, 'You know what, I didn't get done what I needed to get done today and that's okay. That's just what happened today but tomorrow I'll make sure I get that thing done.'

"Taking full responsibility for my own actions and for what I do was huge." He says that when he ends up watching television when he knows he should be doing other, more productive tasks, he doesn't beat himself up or blame himself for not getting things done. Being hard on himself doesn't do any good; rather, he recognizes that he drifted off and tells himself he'll do a much better job the next day.

 ## INNOVATION IN TECHNOLOGY

When Spencer was just thirteen years old, his mother got a smartphone for him because he was always interested in technology. He had to pay for his service plan, and he had to find a way to pay her back for the phone itself. But in the end, it turned out to be an excellent investment. He started making videos on the smartphone and reviewing apps and other technology. To his surprise, he got over one million views in the first month.

"It was such a great thing for a kid with ADHD, because with videos I had to be spontaneous. I didn't have a script." He could make videos when he wanted to make them, and he was having a blast. "I had no problem focusing on them. When I wanted to do something I loved, I had no problem doing it."

This love of technology, apps, and videos was the precursor to a career in technology. He says that, in many cases, the videos took off, and he was asked by several companies to review their apps for his videos. Many of them, according to Spencer, were not very good products. These apps didn't work the way they said they would work; they were ugly, unintuitive, and many even crashed. Spencer was not impressed by many of them.

The frustration Spencer felt in reviewing these inferior products led him to begin creating his own apps. Spencer found voids in the marketplace and began to innovate to solve issues that people had through apps. His first app was based on a very simple concept: backing up your phone and the existing apps on it. At the time, experts considered Spencer's product a must-have. In no time it was downloaded over 40,000 times by users, which sparked his interest in creating more apps and technology.

Spencer's next app was called "Do It." It was a productivity app. You may be surprised that an ADHD guy created a productivity app, but that's exactly what he did. "I always wanted to be around productivity. I always wanted to help people get things done more quickly because that was my biggest thing," he explains. Spencer tries to solve the issue of those with and without ADHD: time management.

The Do It app sat on the desktop of your computer, and you could set reminders with it. After the set time, whether it was ten or twenty minutes or whatever you set it to, the computer screen would flash with your next task. The app could also open up a program, so if you needed to send an email to a colleague, it would open up your email program automatically. The application, in essence, helped people avoid distractions between tasks and helped them stay on track to do the things they needed to get done. At the time, it ended up being a top ten best-selling productivity app.

His next application was a pill-remind app, and that also did very well. It ended up being another top seller in the medical app category for about one year. The project was inspired by his father, who used to forget to take his medication.

Spencer finally made the decision to go to college and, after one semester, decided it wasn't for him and left. He ended up at a technology company in California and eventually was teamed up with a mentor who was a venture capitalist. The venture capitalist mentored him on the business side of technology. After a two-month trip to Europe with a friend, Spencer came back and got a job at a very large technology company in Santa Barbara, California, taking responsibility for user experience for mobile and desktop applications.

Spencer was thrilled to have this opportunity. He was in charge of an incredibly important issue: user experience. What could be more important than the user's experience when it comes to software and computer applications? He cared deeply about it and was able to contribute to some of the design and interfaces that these applications used.

But in true ADHD fashion, he decided after several months that it was time for him to start his own company. He quickly raised $1 million, found a partner who was also in the business, and began to assemble his own team for his software company.

Spencer and his partner began to develop software to help people keep track of their life, circling back to Spencer's earlier fascination with tackling his own problem with time management and scheduling. It's called WeDo, and it's meant to assist you in running your life. You can use it for any part of your life: family, work, and more. In short, the software allows you to create sections of your life called tribes. "It's really the simplest way to get things done with the people around you. I use it for my family; I use it for my work; and I use it for my personal things. I have my personal tribe, which is all the things I need to get done for myself. Then I have my work tribe, which I invited all my employees to, and I can chat with them through it. And then I have all the task lists that they assign to me and I assign to them." With this system, everyone can keep each other accountable for staying on track with projects.

"This doesn't just apply to people with ADHD, of course. This really applies to anyone who needs to get things done with other people in their life. What kind of sparked this whole thing was my problem with getting this done with the people I needed to interact with every day.

"That was the hardest part of having ADHD—I always would forget what I needed to get done. I would always forget when it was due or who I needed to get it to. It was just kind of lost in the ether to me." Growing up, Spencer says he was always taking notes but would bring them home, stuffed in his pockets, and never do anything with them.

how he manages today

As you might imagine, launching a new venture requires a ton or work, effort, time, and resources. And that can be trying for someone with ADHD. It all goes back to having that foundation and the idea that if we don't have certain things in place in our lives, the next great idea will be nothing more than that—an idea with no follow-through. Spencer has put in place a number of things in his life to make sure he is successful with his ventures.

In his business, he surrounds himself with the right people. "The biggest thing that helped me with this whole thing was I was able to hire the people who would work the best with me because that's really hard." He says that for those with ADHD, finding people who can think like you but also complement how you think is what makes things work. "The common saying is that you need to get the right people on the right bus in the right seats going in the right direction. And that's been the luxury for me in starting something on my own."

He says that it's less about adapting to a situation and more about creating an environment that adapts to him. And that's a combination of finding the right people and making sure he delegates what needs to be done in the company. "I just keep everything delegated and clean, and I get things done right when they happen because I just know with ADHD that I'm never going to come back to it."

He also tries to keep his to-do list to a manageable number of tasks and tries to limit the number of emails in his inbox as much as possible. Spencer says he is also a fan of self-analyzing and always forcing himself to do better. "I think what happens a lot is people start punishing themselves, and that's not the right thing. People say to themselves, 'Oh you're doing so bad' or 'I can't believe you did that,' instead of saying, 'I know you can do better.'" He says keeping his morale up is a big thing for him.

Spencer notes that if you are going to be successful and try to conquer your ADHD, you have to stay away from the negative connotations that come with the diagnosis. "That's been the number one thing that's helped me keep myself productive," he says.

The second most important way he manages his ADHD is through meditation. He says that many of us get wrapped up in the fact that we have so many things to accomplish that we end up doing nothing. He doesn't go to meditation classes, and he doesn't meditate for hours on end, but he does use small doses of meditation to get through the day. Meditating even in short bursts keeps him from feeling overwhelmed and giving up.

Diet and exercise are very important to him. "If I eat badly or I don't exercise, I can get very unproductive." He says that keeping himself in a good physical state is vital.

"When I was growing up with ADHD, there was nothing really out there about the good side of it. It was always about how to keep it down and how to basically beat it to the ground, not, 'Hey, look at all the great things you can do with it.'"

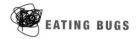

EATING BUGS

Kevin Bachhuber sells bugs. And guess what? You may be eating them. Kevin is the founder of Big Cricket Farms, and he raises and sells crickets to those who eat them. How's that for innovation?

Kevin was born in 1984 and at the age of four was diagnosed with ADHD. While his parents were somewhat resistant to medication, he finally did start taking it for his ADHD. He had a need for movement, and oftentimes he was given a pass in school to get out of the classroom and move around, even though he was taking medication. He always had a mind that wandered, and to this day he says that if meetings go on too long, he begins to drift off and suggests a break.

Always having an entrepreneurial spirit, at six years old he was weeding the gardens of neighbors and earned $65 in one summer. He says he spent it on Legos™.

After his parents divorced, he says life was somewhat chaotic. But he found a comic book store down the street from his house and started to go there often. "It was one of those places that doubled as a store and the cheapest child care you could buy," recalls Kevin. When he turned eighteen, he bought into the store with a combination of cash and $10,000 worth of Magic: The Gathering cards. "I kind of came into my own at that store."

The store gave Kevin a number of opportunities that dovetailed with his ADHD. Kevin was an affable person, so being in a retail operation was a good fit for him. It also offered him the complexity that he craved so he would not get bored. "The store was a really good outlet and template in terms of how I would use ADHD as an advantage, rather than a disadvantage," he says. There were a dozen people who worked there and then a handful of volunteers, so there was always someone there who could do the things that he was not as strong at, such as inventory.

He was doing this while he was in high school, and then he went to college. As he puts it, "That sucked." At the college he attended, Kevin said, there was very little support for people like him, who had ADHD. He said that even note taking was something he struggled with. "It was hard to get any type of support in college." He got a degree in English because he said it was an easy major. He also went to college to prove that he could actually complete a four-year project. "I didn't really have any interest in college, but it was expected."

He didn't think working at the comic book store would actually support him, so right after college he got a job in a bank call center. At the same time, he ended up getting married to a woman who seemed to feel that ADHD was just a symptom of laziness. At her suggestion, he tried to decrease his medication. He did, and that was a bad call. It began to affect him, bringing out old patterns of behavioral issues: in particular, issues with authority.

In the end, Kevin quit his job and got a divorce. He ended up getting a different job in financial services, and that wasn't a good fit, either. "The pay sucked, and it wasn't a good space for me morally, either," he explains.

All the while he was keeping his eyes open for a situation in which he could really put his skills into action and make a difference. He looked at various industries and businesses and then read a United Nations report on how many people from other countries were eating insects as food. It was something that he had read about before, so he was aware of the concept, but he never took action on it. At that time, he was working with his girlfriend, providing IT services to healthcare clients, so they were able to build up a little nest egg, and they used that money to start Big Cricket Farms.

Big Cricket Farms is the first urban cricket farm in the country. Based in Youngstown, Ohio, it gave Kevin the opportunity to set two goals: (1) to build this business from the ground up and (2) to strengthen the economic revitalization of the area. The farm is housed in an old warehouse that seems like the last place for a farm of any kind but is actually an ideal location. Before reading the UN report, Kevin had already visited Thailand and sampled crickets himself. He had even entertained the idea of cricket farming before he read the UN report, but when he found no initial interest, he had shelved it. It wasn't until the UN document became popular that he decided to take the plunge.

As you can imagine, Kevin's business has enjoyed all kinds of media attention and was even featured on CNN. Because the business is unique, it has caught the attention of many in the media. That media attention has helped boost awareness of the business as well as sales.

At any given time, Big Cricket Farms is raising about five thousand pounds of crickets. And they are well on their way to raising one billion crickets a year. Kevin's business is strictly wholesale, meaning he supplies the crickets to food companies and distributors, and they in turn, market these to various stores, such as health food stores and restaurants. They also supply companies that use the bugs to make protein powders. Kevin has even created partnerships with other cricket farms to help supply pet stores and other operations. Since Kevin started Big Cricket Farms, other similar companies have popped up, so you might say he started a revolution in the bug-eating trend that is starting to crawl across the country.

Kevin thinks there are a number of factors in ADHD that dovetail with entrepreneurship. He says that the energy that comes with being ADHD plays well, especially in the start-up world. The hours can be long when starting a new company, so that energy can be an asset.

"Creativity is key to coming up with something that's distinctive from anything around it," Kevin adds. That has certainly been the case in his experience. He has also managed to leverage his affable personality into valuable publicity for his business. He says he is a guy who likes to talk and having reporters interview him has satisfied that urge. While he was in school, he may have been criticized for talking too much, but these days it's an essential skill that has benefited him in many ways.

Also, he says, owning his own business is great because he never does anything the same way twice. As he admits, "I'm just incapable of doing it. And that works out very well with the press, because I'm never telling the same story twice. Each [journalist] walks away with a little different story that examines different aspects of this large complex thing."

He also says that you need to live your life in accordance with how your brain functions. He mentions that youngsters can get on an Individualized Education Plan (IEP) at school and get extra help, but when you get out of school and start working, the real world is unlikely to make accommodations for you because you have ADHD. The message here is that you should choose your career and business carefully and make sure you can be of value. Any human being wants to leverage her strengths, and people with ADHD are no different.

Leveraging your ADHD also means trying to find out what you are good at and applying your unique skills to a career or business idea. Brendan Mahan, whom we met in chapter 3, says that even though people with ADHD need things to change on occasion, that is not such a bad thing. "The fact that we tend to get bored more easily means that we tend to push the envelope and get things done because we want to be productive and we want to be moving forward. Brendan goes on to say that people with ADHD are generally good at starting things and fixing things. "Go into a career where that's what you're doing," says Brendan.

"Accounting is not usually a good career for people with ADHD because it's kind of the same thing over and over again. It's not a new and interesting problem that you need to solve." If you have ADHD and enjoy your career in accounting, it's likely you've found a way to see what you do each day as a new challenge, so this isn't a prescription for everyone—it's all about perspective. That said, if your job emphasizes consistency and repetition, it might present difficulties for you if you have ADHD.

Entrepreneurship is a natural fit for those with ADHD, says Brendan, because, for the most part, it's about "starting things and fixing stuff." And when we begin to find certain tasks difficult or no longer fun, entrepreneurs are free to hire someone to help us out. "When it gets slow and tedious, hire someone who can do the slow and tedious stuff so you can refocus on what you are good at, which is vision, drive, and ideas," Brendan suggests.

Working for yourself is not for everyone, whether or not you have ADHD. There's no way to generalize: We are not all destined to become business owners, nor do we all lack an appetite for authority. We are not all software programmers at heart. But many of us with ADHD do go on to find a career that they can be good at and maintain an interest in, and that chosen career may be in one of many fields. Those of us with ADHD are not unlike anyone else. We try to find something we love, and if we don't feel fulfilled or satisfied, we move on. We may, however, move on a little more abruptly than others.

What many of those with ADHD do fall into are high-energy and intense careers. "Entrepreneurship is not the only place for people with ADHD to be successful. People with ADHD tend to be very good in the military or real good as fireman or police officers or EMTs, because when everything goes crazy we tend to get calm," says Brendan. It just happens to be the opposite for those without ADHD. Adults with ADHD may tend to be kind of fuzzy in the brain in normal situations, but when chaos breaks out, many of us suddenly take control of the situation. Those without ADHD may be "clearer" on a day-to-day basis, but when a crisis occurs, they lose control. Still, everyone is different—just don't discount your ability to stay cool in emotionally charged situations and find solutions on the fly. If you love high-intensity work, find a career or a business that you can apply your crisis management skills to. When you find a career or a business that allows you to constantly be in the zone, you've won.

Brendan concludes, saying, "Put some work into figuring out what your ideal working environment is. If you're really weak with people but good with patterns and systems, maybe computer programming is [for you]. On the other hand if you are gregarious but can't put two lines together on a spreadsheet, maybe customer service is right for you. You have to look for a job that fits you and not just a job that you can get."

As for the cricket business, Kevin feels that he found his calling and that he'll be doing it for at least ten years. "It's custom-fit for me: It's complex; it involves talking with a lot of people; there's a lot of moving parts; and there are constantly shifting opportunities." He says insect farming is a fast and emerging market. "It's ideally suited for my need for speed and my need to not be bored."

The moral of the story? Once you have gained an understanding of your unique strengths and weaknesses, go out and find what you are good at and what nourishes your soul.

a solid support system

Almost anyone who has experienced any kind of lasting success has some type of support system in his life. That support has a hand in your business life, and it certainly needs to be in your personal life. Some people need an incredible amount of support and assistance, while others just need a good nudge every now and then. Most people with ADHD I talked with had some type of support or mentoring in their lives. And while some people just have an epiphany and find a way to chart a course on their own, most have people around them and systems that allow them to be successful with their ADHD.

Even if you are a small business owner and you hire the right people to help you in your business, you are creating a support system that works for you. Socially, even if your support system is a Meetup group of adults with ADHD, finding something that allows you to have positive people around you keeps you from getting down about your ADHD. The only tricky thing is finding the right ways to build that network in a way that works with who you are as a person.

Dr. Hallowell emphasizes the concept of finding the right support. "Marry the right person, and find the right job," says

Dr. Hallowell. You need to find the right personal support and the right partners in your life. "You need someone with attention surplus disorder," he says. "You need the people who can count the beans and make the trains run on time." Dr. Hallowell says that almost never is anyone with ADHD successful on her own. "It's the right collaboration that makes the big difference."

The people who get into trouble with their ADHD and end up spinning their wheels are the ones who reject any help at all. And while Dr. Hallowell doesn't like the term "accountability," he does stress the importance of goals and making sure that you are meeting them. "We come up with the ideas—the ADD people are the idea factories. We're always generating ideas. But implementation—that's where we have trouble, and that's where we need help."

ADHD coach Brendan Mahan echoes these comments. "It's really important to have a good partner," says Brendan. And that goes for both home and work or business. "You want to have a partner who has strong executive functioning skills. Just having a strong partner who has those skills is going to help you be successful, whether it's in business or family."

"We need a lot of support," says ADHD coach Dana Rayburn. She says that it is important to have someone to help you out and be that sounding board or, as she describes it, your scaffolding. She says that person needs to help us stick to our goals and plans as well as be realistic about what we are up to. Dana does use the word "accountability," and she thinks it's important to have someone like herself by your side to keep you on track. She says that many with ADHD are like that birthday balloon in your house that is untethered—it just floats around aimlessly until it deflates. "We need someone to hold onto that string and keep us moving in the direction we want to move in."

Dana adds, "I also think we need support because we tend to be people who are better when we have other energy, and we're more focused and able to get things done when we have someone else around." She says, in essence, it's great to have that body double to give us a nudge and positive energy to keep us moving forward. I completely agree. When I go to a meeting with other business owners and energetic businesspeople, I get really motivated to do better. The energy is definitely contagious. I used to belong to business networking groups that met at 7 a.m., and while I hated going there, once I got there I was full of energy because I was so inspired by the people around me.

We met Chris Berlow earlier in this book. While he is not an ADHD-specific coach, he has many years of experience in helping people live up to their potential, both in his martial arts business and as an empowerment coach. He is very astute at helping people figure out the things in their lives that are blocking success, as well as helping people set and achieve goals.

"Athletes at the elite level have coaches," says Chris. And while that coach does have a certain expertise and knowledge, she is also there to make sure the athlete is doing the work that he needs to do to excel and win. "People in general think that they can handle it on their own, but there is no better way to raise up your level than to have someone hold you accountable."

Chris also feels that, for an entrepreneur, coaching is vital, because it allows you to move toward the path of working *on* your business and not *in* the business all the time. And we know that those with ADHD can get bogged down in some of the more laborious tasks of running a business and that can lead to dissatisfaction and ultimately getting nothing done. Your business or career can't grow unless you are spending time working on it. And proper support is vital to making that happen.

Like many of our fellow humans, we don't always ask for help. However, those of us with ADHD need to be open to having that support system around us. Chris feels that there is a certain amount of pride that gets in the way of asking for help. "Somebody with an open mind and a willingness to look at new ways of doing things is going to be the one who is more successful."

Dana Rayburn agrees that many people with ADHD don't always ask for help, and that can be tough if your life gets out of control before you do ask for that help. "I think there is a lot of resistance, and by the time people come to me, they have hit the wall and they have to change." She says that oftentimes it gets to the point when a person with ADHD is in jeopardy of losing his job or his marriage is falling apart. That's when he finally calls Dana or some other ADHD coach or professional. Frustration has set in, and he acknowledges that he needs help.

"I think typical people just muddle along and think they can do it and don't get the help that they need for whatever reason. They don't think they deserve it, or they don't want it, or they think they can do things on their own," Dana notes. Yes, many of us have been successful without a coach or mentor, but it can take longer when you go it alone. Getting someone like Dana or one of the other ADHD coaches you met in this book can be an enormous asset in your life. "Hit the easy button, for Christ sake," says Dana. "Get stuff done and get it done fast because it doesn't have to be so hard."

Most successful people, whether they have ADHD or not, have a good support system, including a coach or a mentor. Having someone who keeps you on track and can help you set and achieve goals as well as help you get past your perceptions of your limitations is well worth your time. "Most people do better when we have got someone else external pulling us forward. My job as a coach is to teach them the skills so they can go off and do it on their own. I want them to learn the skills, I want them to learn to be self-sufficient so they go off and do what they need to do on their own," Dana says.

Dana and other coaches have regular clients they have seen for years. Her ADHD clients benefit from that regular check-in with her. If you have a call coming up with your coach, Dana feels that's a good deadline. What might make an ADHD coach a little different from an executive coach is that he might have a greater understanding of the underlying causes of why you may have struggled with deadlines in the past. And if you don't make a certain deadline, then you can work together to figure out why and work toward meeting the next one without being shamed and blamed for not getting something done. If you are concerned that a general life coach may not understand your unique issues, look for one who will get who you are. "We are so used to being blamed and ashamed for so much in our lives. And ADHD coaching is this place where it's just really safe to just be who you are and it's okay." Dana says it's important to have someone by your side who understands why you do the things you do and what makes you tick.

But hiring a coach and then not putting that advice into action is a waste of your time and money. Working with a coach takes a commitment from you to make sure you can put in the time and energy to change. You don't have to become this incredible super-productive person overnight, but you do need to come to the table with a willingness to at least make the small changes that are necessary. Dana suggests making sure you do what your coach says and listen very carefully. She also suggests that you make time immediately after your coaching call or appointment to try to get some of the items you discussed on your call done, if you can. Many of us end our coaching calls and don't get to our to-do list until right before the next call. She says that by setting aside time directly after the call to work on your coaching items, you'll feel less anxiety about completing them before your next appointment.

Dana also says it's important for you to pay close attention, and not just while you're on the call. She recommends making sure you are paying attention to how you are feeling, what you are thinking, how you are acting, and just generally maintaining a sense of where you are in the world. Cultivating awareness is huge, she says, because without that self-awareness we can't make adjustments. You hired a coach to help you make key changes in your life, so there is no doubt that you'll be going through some emotional upheavals during the process. Dana says that many make the mistake of not listening to this advice, and it just won't work well unless you listen to your coach and work things through.

You should also consider an ADHD coach if you are having issues at work. If you are on some type of corrective action plan, as they might call it in the corporate world, and you think that your ADHD is causing you not to do well at your job, you should look into working with someone who specializes in ADHD coaching. They can help you create the tools you need to get back on track and offer you advice on dealing with your employer or boss. If you don't tackle this issue head-on, you could lose your job and jeopardize future employment.

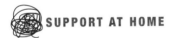 SUPPORT AT HOME

Coaching will work if you put your mind to it, but you also need to make sure that if you are married or have a significant other that he or she offers you support as well. Your own personal ADHD chaos is not confined to your workplace; it's also in the home. And you need support and understanding there as well. Dana says that your spouse can and should be one of your biggest supporters. "They need to learn as much as they can about ADHD, and they really need to be able to accept and love that their spouse is doing the absolute best that they can and that they are trying the best that they can. Everybody has stuff they need to deal with, and with ADD, our stuff is much more apparent so the spouse just needs to be patient, needs to be understanding, needs to help keep the support system in place and not get frustrated."

Melissa Orlov is a marriage consultant as well as a top authority on the subject of how ADHD affects relationships. She also cowrites the blog *ADHD and Marriage* with Dr. Hallowell and is the author of two books, *The ADHD Effect on Marriage* (Specialty Press, 2010) and *The Couples Guide to Thriving with ADHD* (Specialty Press, 2014). She says it is critical to have that external support system. "It's important to create these external structures simply because the mind of the person who has ADHD is pretty energetic and fairly disorganized because of the kinds of information coming in and the lack of filters on that information and the fact that it is not naturally hierarchical," which, she points out, is a benefit of ADHD in some situations, but not in others.

Most people come to see Melissa because they are struggling with their relationship. She points out that many are actually doing very well in their business or their place of work when things begin to fall apart at home, where there is no structure unless you create it. She contends that the lack of structure in the personal relationship tends to manifest itself as inconsistency. Inconsistency, in turn, makes you seem unreliable, and that leads to a lack of trust. "In the workplace that sort of gets covered by the structures and the time lines and deadlines and all the things that are in the calendar, but at home, not so much. And as soon as you lose trust in your partner, then you have lost a great deal. So that's why creating these structures is so important." Melissa goes on to say that creating structures in the home leads to trust between partners.

What you need to be careful of, according to Melissa, is having an imbalance in your relationship at home. If the non-ADHD partner is required to create that structure, the relationship becomes imbalanced; so, in essence, they are no longer partners on the same level. If one person creates the structure and requires the ADHD person to adhere to that, it can result in the parent-child dynamic, and that doesn't work in a relationship. If you are not involved in the process of creating that structure in the home—that is, someone else has done it for you—you can start to be treated like a child or a less important person, and that is no way to create a working support system. In short, you need to be part of the solution to make this work.

Now there is no evidence that ADHD is contagious, but if you as the ADHD person do not place some of your own structures in the home or in your relationship, your issues can have an impact on your spouse. If your spouse has to pick up the slack for your lack of organization or inability to get things done, that can become overwhelming for her. It's not that she acquires ADHD, but rather that managing your issues on top of her own can cause negative effects in her life.

Melissa describes a scenario in which the ADHD person is responsible for picking up the kids from school and, on a regular basis, forgets or is late. Then the school calls, wondering where the parent is. Not only are the kids stranded, but now you have inconvenienced the school staff as well, since a teacher or administrator will need to watch them until one of the parents finally gets there. After a number of these types of situations, your spouse begins to wonder every day when the other shoe is going to drop. He has no idea whether you are going to forget to pick up the kids again, and he has to be constantly "on" in order to react quickly to your disorganization. Not only that, but then he begins to regularly check in on you, and that leads to incredible stress and resentment.

So, as the ADHD person in the relationship, you need to be able to create structure in your home life so you can be a reliable partner. Melissa amends this statement and says that you just have to be "reliable enough." Because of who you are as an ADHD adult, you will probably need a backup system, and your partner needs to be willing and able to adapt to that. But if the issue continues to arise and your partner is always covering for you, you need to sit down and fix the problem.

Notice, so far, that this has not been about everyone supporting you with you putting in no effort. Yes, you need as much support as you can get as a person with ADHD, but just because you have support doesn't mean you can put in less effort yourself. You need to have people around you, both at home and in your business life, who understand you and can support you, but they will only do so if you have skin in the game.

In terms of your partner or spouse, it is very important for both of you to have a full understanding of what ADHD is and what it is to you specifically, according to Melissa. "I think the number one issue if you've had any problems at all is for both partners to get a very full understanding of ADHD and what I call the ADHD effect." She advises not to totally define your life around ADHD, but for the purpose of being able to understand it and find out why certain patterns are there in your life, you need to understand its most noticeable features, both in a diagnostic sense and in terms of your unique personality. She goes on to say that once you understand your ADHD, you then have access to a whole host of tools that can help you with that support system.

She also says it's crucial for both of you to accept that you have ADHD. You have to get out of denial and face the fact that ADHD is in your life. Maybe it's there and you both deal with it, but there can also be anger and frustration on both sides, and those emotions need to be acknowledged and dealt with. She recommends getting out of mutual denial, if it exists. "Having ADHD in your relationship really does matter because it has the potential to hit at the heart of your relationship."

Melissa says that once you both develop a mutual understanding and acceptance of ADHD in your lives, you can begin to focus on the positives.

She also says that a good partner for someone who has ADHD is a person who understands ADHD, who has the ability to let certain things go by in the moment and not let issues stick with him, but also has the courage to go to you and address that issue before it gets out of hand if he sees a pattern emerging. Of course, this should be done in a gentle and thoughtful way. Your partner should be able to listen and be empathetic, and that needs to go both ways. As a person with ADHD, you need to have the same qualities when dealing with conflict.

Melissa says you both need to practice what is called "conflict intimacy." Whether you have ADHD in your life or not, the best way to resolve conflict in your life is to do so with a level of respect and restraint. You need to cultivate an ability to speak nonaggressively and listen without getting defensive immediately. She says you have to have those qualities and those skill sets in your relationship. "It takes a fair amount of perseverance in any marriage, regardless of whether ADHD is there, and I think particularly when you have ADHD there, because of the inconsistencies you come up against."

Your partner also needs to be patient. Things may not change as fast as you'd like them to because of your ADHD symptoms, so Melissa says that not only does your partner have to be empathic to that, but she also must be as patient as she can be. A good sense of humor will go a long way in an ADHD relationship. You have to be able to laugh at it sometimes. Yes, forgetting to pick up your children at school might not be something you can laugh at, but other situations just need humor injected in them sometimes. Being serious about your ADHD all the time will get you nowhere.

So how do you start the conversation with your partner if you haven't done so already? Melissa says it's important for you, the person with ADHD, to have a little self-reflection. The temptation is to go to your partner and tell him what he is doing wrong or to blame him for certain things going on. That clearly won't work, and it's a big inhibiter to having an open and constructive conversation. She says that you need to ask yourself how seriously you are taking your ADHD and even ask if you have gotten an official diagnosis. Perhaps it's worth visiting a medical professional to determine whether your problems are specific to ADHD or if you might be dealing with other challenges that a medical professional can help you through. Reexamine if you have been taking care of yourself and getting the proper treatment and other support you need. Go back to chapter 4 on creating a solid foundation.

"Before you go to your partner, make sure you are taking your ADHD seriously," Melissa says. When you approach your partner to discuss a problem, make sure you acknowledge that it is a two-way issue. Do not blame your spouse or significant other; rather, state the fact that there is a problem, and identify the fact that it needs to be addressed jointly.

Just because you might be having issues in your relationship right now, you can still make it work. But just like any relationship, you have to keep working at it. "People need to understand that even if their relationship is in pretty bad shape right now, and the chances are better than not that it is, that is not an indication of whether or not they can have a good relationship in the future." Melissa says that there will likely be issues in a relationship. "Once you do know what's going on in a relationship, you really can turn it around, so it's really imperative to get educated about this, and there's a great outcome if you do usually." She says you can learn how to thrive and that a great support system in your partner is not as far away as you think it might be. Melissa recommends being hopeful and putting the time and energy into this.

Both of you have a great deal of influence on how your relationship will continue and thrive with ADHD in the mix. If you have not done your part in managing your ADHD, getting treatment, and getting serious about it, don't expect your partner to pick up the slack without you showing him that you are ready to make a difference. Melissa says that using your ADHD as an excuse is not an option and that you need to be fully engaged. Men, in particular, tend to disengage, and she says that you cannot disengage and have a relationship that works. If you are truly committed, find a way to engage with your partner constructively.

You should also take the time to go on the website Melissa shares with Dr. Hallowell. You can find that blog at https://www.adhdmarriage.com. Not only will you find great information on this subject, but there is also a wealth of tools available to you. You'll also have access to her couples seminar that is held by phone.

I can't help you find the right husband or wife—that's totally up to you. But my advice when looking for any type of external support is to find those you feel comfortable with and who are a good fit for your needs. I have not used an ADHD coach, but I have used other coaches that have helped me immensely in my life and business. It had to be a good fit, and I needed to respect that person as someone who could truly help me, understand me, and work together with me to help me get where I needed to be.

CHAPTER ELEVEN

find your way

Some of the greatest success I discovered with individuals with ADHD came from the greatest adversity. So if you are the type of person who needs to see how others found their way in life despite a few obstacles put up in their way, you'll want to meet the individuals here.

One person cited in this book needed to remain anonymous, and that is "Michael B." Michael is a very successful man in the investment business, but his road to success was anything but easy. At times, it got pretty scary.

"Growing up I never really felt like I fit in. I felt like I was a little bit different from other kids, and like a lot of people with ADHD, I was smart enough to just power through not doing homework," says Michael. He says that despite messing around in class and being very impulsive, he got through school. "I always underperformed relative to where I thought I should, and looking back now, I think it had a pretty significant emotional effect on me."

He never did homework, and never wanted to do homework, but when he really got interested in something he could hyperfocus for days. He played piano as a kid, and when he didn't like a piece of music, he wouldn't practice, but when he did come across a piece of music he found appealing, he would work on it for days. He also played golf competitively as a kid. "If I enjoyed eighteen holes, I wanted to play fifty-four and not stop until I was exhausted."

He remembers that in freshman-year biology in high school he got a D-plus, and his mother was called in to school for a conference. The teacher gave him the "get your act together" speech and moved on. He aced the next three exams due to the pressure. "It wasn't a question of ability, it was a question of willingness and ability to sit down and stay focused on my own." He was actually surprised at how well he could do when he applied himself, but unfortunately, he didn't apply himself going forward.

Michael got through high school, but he feels that this started a pattern of lying to cover up his mistakes and a lack of willingness to do assignments, which became an important aspect in his life later on. He says he lied to his parents and teachers and tried to be manipulative to get away with not doing homework and other assignments. "I was just smart and charming enough to pull it off." He feels that lying and overcompensating for gaps in ability and focus can cause a lot of shame in ADHD people.

By his senior year in high school, Michael finally did get into college, and he thought to himself that he had the worst case of undiagnosed ADHD, because he always acted just a little crazy. At the time, he just had a suspicion that he had ADHD, but he did not get diagnosed and was not on medication at that point.

He was accepted by a pretty good college in the UK, despite his setbacks in high school. Many students from the United States went to this school, and because the academic standards for Americans were a bit lower (perhaps because they paid full tuition), he got in. "If I could bullshit my way on an essay, which I did, I could kind of manipulate them into letting me in, and they did."

He still didn't have a diagnosis, because he feels he was very good at manipulating and putting on a good face. He also felt that everyone saw him as someone who had nothing wrong with him, and he felt that eventually he would get his act together as he grew up.

So he got to college in the UK, partied a lot, and had a great time, but didn't do a whole lot of work. He had some success in school, but all in all he underperformed and came back home after his freshman year. He said to himself again that he must have ADHD and began the process of getting tested. The test proved that he did have ADHD, and he was prescribed Adderall after his freshman year. "My world changed dramatically."

"When I took Adderall, it gave me motivation, so I just needed to wait for it to kick in, and then I would get motivated to do something, as opposed to having to generate that organically." He was taking the prescribed amount of Adderall and was motivated to get a tutor and work hard to get good grades. He said math was never his strong suit, but as he studied financial economics and advanced algebra, his working memory got better. "My grades went through the roof. I felt like this is it—this is what I've been missing, and this is going to help me become my best self. I loved it, and it worked for a while."

He said that there were probably some warning signs in the beginning that he regrets not paying attention to, but being on medication helped him with tasks and organization that he always lacked. "I felt like I could compete intellectually with anybody. It made me feel like Superman. It was that dramatic of an experience at first."

But Michael began to use his medication for the wrong reasons. He says that it was working to help him get through classes and his day, and then he would go out at night. He would wake up the next morning and be tired, so he would take medication to essentially keep himself awake. "I started to use it as a crutch for energy instead of what it was prescribed for."

Entering his senior year at college, he was taking extended-release medication as well as instant-release pills. He started having myoclonic jerks, which are not so much seizures but are more involuntary muscle twitches. They got so bad that he had to take his senior year off. He spent the next several months going to doctors to try to discover what was wrong with him. He feels that after testing, which showed nothing, that he began to abuse his medication in earnest. Then, when he stopped taking his medication for a brief period, the jerks seemed to vanish.

He got back to the UK to finish up his senior year and things began to unravel again. He actually had a job lined up already but stopped caring about classes at that point. He started his medication again and at that point was taking double the amount he had been taking before.

Michael did get a degree, but not in finance as he wanted. He didn't complete his dissertation, so he was not eligible for his degree in finance and received a liberal arts degree only. "By the end of that year, I could not even write an email. Instead of helping me get organized and be articulate, it [the medication] did the opposite and started to turn on me."

He came home, took a couple months off, and started a job in a financial firm. He had a great relationship with the owner of the firm, who even became Michael's mentor. And that's where Michael says his medication use went through the roof and his life started to go off the rails. He was doing international trading for the firm, which meant he had to stay up at different hours of the day to accommodate trading in other parts of the world, such as Asia. And he was taking his medication at that point to keep himself energized and awake.

He was abusing the drug to the point where he would take a pill, stay in bed until it started working, and then he would get up. "It never felt like I was chasing a feeling, it just felt like I was doing what I needed to do to be a successful professional." He said he was never chasing a high—he just wanted to do well and keep up. At this point, Michael believes he was taking much more medication to get the same effect. "I started to have to take a lot of Adderall just to get out and function for the day." Michael also states that, at this point in his life, he had no other strategies to deal with or manage his ADHD.

Now his life fell into complete disarray. He says that the medication stopped working and helping him to do the things he was taking it for in the first place. He stopped paying his bills, even though he had the money; he let his auto insurance lapse; his apartment turned into a primal state of squalor, with layers of trash and other belongings scattered all over the place. While he points out that he is certainly not proud of what he has told me so far, he feels that it's important for people to know. At least to the people at work, he seemed to have his act together, so no one had an indication of what was going on with him.

He would even go upwards of a week living on diet cola and coffee and maybe binge eat on the weekend. By this time his apartment and car were both so stuffed with trash that he stopped talking to friends. He even skipped a friend's wedding.

One night he put a cigarette out in his car and went to bed only to find out that the cigarette hadn't actually been extinguished. The inside of his garbage-stuffed car caught on fire in the parking lot and blew out the windshield. At this point his father became concerned, so he drove out to check on him and found Michael in this state.

It took Michael's father a week to clean out his apartment, and after that, Michael checked into a rehabilitation facility. "Thank God I was able to keep my ears open long enough to understand that I had a problem." He spent three months in the rehab facility and then eight months in a halfway house to get better. He spent a total of eleven months getting his life back together, and then it was time to get back to work.

He teamed up with a partner he had worked with in his previous firm and set out to get his life back, starting a new financial services firm. Michael runs the investment side of the business, and his partner is in charge of the financial planning part of the company. At the time of the publication of this book, they had about $50 million under management for clients and growing. In essence, Michael is the portfolio manager. He also runs a discretionary macro hedge fund. He is dealing with both individual retirement plans and some high-net-worth clients. His partner understands him and his ADHD, and they can be totally honest with each other.

Michael is becoming that successful person he always wanted to be, but now he needs to put a number of things in place in his life to ensure that he doesn't slip back to where he was. He hired someone to come in and clean his apartment once a week and to cook various meals for him. That was one of his first steps. He feels that in college you are supposed to learn how to be a professional and keep your life in order, but that didn't happen for him. He let his medication manage his life.

It may be second nature to many without ADHD, but Michael manages his professional life through a combination of his Outlook calendar and a notebook. At night he reviews what he needs to get done the next day at work and does that again in the morning. Like so many of the other people interviewed for this book, he says that staying on routine is absolutely critical.

What Michael calls "batching," along with being "in the zone," is vital to getting through a day as well. By batching, he means that he saves the task of emailing people and other tasks that can throw him off track and does these all at once, sometimes waiting a couple days to respond to all his emails. By being in the zone, he means that he has to be in the right frame of mind to perform during the trading day. "I try to put myself in a position where I can do market analysis and trade and kind of be in the cockpit without any other extraneous distractions." He doesn't have his email program up during the day, and he tells his assistant that he is off-limits unless a matter is critical. "I don't let anybody into my world during that period so I can focus on what I'm doing." He says he has to function that way because he knows that it doesn't take much to drastically alter the course of how his day is going.

He has hired the right people as well, including someone who can compile data and reports for him. "Operating day-to-day for me is tough, and it goes against my nature, so I've surrounded myself with people who can help me fit into that box." That box allows Michael to stay in the zone and do what he does best, which is to analyze data and make sound investment decisions. ADHD was crippling to Michael for many years of his life, but he has now turned this negative into a positive and leverages his ADHD qualities to help him build his business.

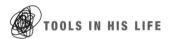 **TOOLS IN HIS LIFE**

Aside from keeping his work and home environment tight and controlled, Michael does a number of things to feed his inner drive and soul. One thing he relies on in his life is meditation, not medication. Part of his morning and afternoon routine involves practicing transcendental meditation. He took a class, and at first, he admits he was not sold on the idea, but he also admits that it changed him in the long term. "It ended up being one of the best things I've ever done. It dramatically improves my focus and my clarity of thought." He says that if people with ADHD don't want to do any other work for themselves, he would recommend meditation above any other activity. He feels that it is one of the few things that had a profound effect on his life after medication. He likes hiking, too, and being out in the wilderness has helped him as well.

Michael also stopped almost all of his social media consumption. "I got off pretty much all social media about two years ago: Facebook, LinkedIn, the works. Everything except Twitter, which I use in a limited capacity for news and financial markets–related things that relate to my job. An honest, objective appraisal of my social media habits revealed I was using them compulsively, and they provided too easy an immediate gratification distraction from whatever I wanted to be focusing on. I make an effort to keep in touch with friends and family via email, Skype, and by telephone. Our communication is richer as a result."

He has also created boundaries in his use of the Internet. "I use the Stay Focused productivity browser extension on Google Chrome. I have pretty much everything not work related blocked with the 'Nuclear Options,' which is irreversible. The first few weeks using it I found myself trying to go to some of these sites in a Pavlovian fashion, but eventually settled down, and it's really done its job helping me keep on task.

"I'm the happiest and clearest I've ever been, and it took going through all that to get here."

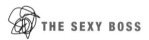 **THE SEXY BOSS**

Heather Ann Havenwood describes herself as a serial entrepreneur. She has started a number of successful businesses, has a popular podcast, and serves as a successful sales and marketing coach for many business professionals. She also runs some very successful dating and coaching businesses that to this day are thriving.

Fast-forward to the end of our call: She said that one of her favorite quotes ends with the phrase, "I'm exactly where I want to be in my life." She is satisfied to report that she does feel that way herself. But as you'll find out, that was not always the case.

Heather was diagnosed with ADHD as a small child but, as she says, she was not actually hyper. She feels she was more of an introvert, but very sensitive, even hypersensitive, to her surroundings. Her mother felt there might be something a little different about Heather, so they scheduled a doctor visit, and she was ultimately diagnosed with ADHD. Her primary doctor prescribed Ritalin. She didn't completely understand why she was taking it at that time.

Her mother enrolled her in a private school where the class size was small, and Heather feels that worked and that is an environment in which she felt comfortable. She does remember one day in second grade when she did not take her medication. She heard everything but what the teacher was saying. "The teacher is up at the front, and I can't hear the teacher. I hear the ball outside; I hear this kid tapping his foot; I hear a kid tapping his pencil; and I hear everything except the teacher. I felt like I wanted to scream."

She ended up back in public school because the private school was too expensive. She started speech therapy, and it was somewhat interesting that she spent time there, because much of what she does now involves speaking.

In school she had challenges with reading comprehension and writing, and actually failed second-grade spelling. But Heather says she was great at math. "You give me something to solve, and I'm good. Give me something to memorize, I hated it." If she had to stand up in front of the class and give a book report, she hated that as well. She just could not get what was in her head out. "I think that's one of the things with ADHD—the mind is going faster than the whole room. I see everybody; I know what's going on in the room; I feel everything; I feel the energy in the room; I see the dynamics, but I don't know what to do with that."

Her escape during those years was ballet. She then got into dance and drill team in high school, and she feels these activities were her outlets. She says she was always into fitness, and the times in her life when she let those activities go were the times where she felt the worst.

She went off to college and promptly flunked out. She then enrolled in a smaller college and did well there. "I think it was because it was like the private school—very small and intimate and there were only thirty people in the class." She feels that this setting was much more interactive and calm. She ended up getting a lot of A's in her classes. She transferred and ultimately attended another small university in Texas, taking classes at night where class sizes were small, and she continued to do well. She earned her degree with a minor in math.

Heather worked various jobs after college, and as she says, she got fired from just about every one of them. "I don't do well in companies, I don't do well in the structure of 'You must do this' and 'You have to do it this way.'" When she hires people in her own company now, she gives them a challenge and tells them to go solve it, because that's what she likes to do.

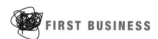 **FIRST BUSINESS**

Heather's first venture was a real estate business. She had a partner, and they grew revenue to over $1 million in just twelve months. Things were going great until she went away for a weekend seminar. She returned to the office on Monday only to find the office completely cleaned out. Not only that, but passwords had been changed, merchant and bank account numbers had been changed, and everything she had worked for was gone. In 2005, she declared bankruptcy and spent the next two years cleaning that mess up.

Before this happened, she had the attitude that nothing could stop her. She was doing well, and her business was growing rapidly, but she says this was the event that crashed her life. "Here I am at the age of thirty-one, and I am bankrupt." After moving away for a year and, as she puts it, staring off into space, the idea-generating side of her ADHD kicked in again, and she decided it was time to get her creativity back. "That was a key piece and I needed that. I think that's a key piece of ADHD—we're creators. If we're not creating something, that's where we get bored."

She created her first business, and yes, her business partner walked away with it, but she felt it was time to create again. She moved back to Austin, Texas, and started an online dating business called Dating Triggers, where she teaches men how to date women. She had a lot of online marketing experience, so it was a great business for her to start. It was also important for her to build something that no one could question her on. She was single and dating men, and she felt she had a lot of advice she could offer them. And she certainly wasn't going back into the real estate business in 2008.

Things were going very well, and from there, Heather wrote the book *Sexy Boss* after getting the idea from a friend. The friend said to her one day, "You know, you are kind of like the 'sexy boss.'" Her friend felt that she was a very good-looking woman, she liked to be in charge, had great ideas, and that the potential brand of empowering people, especially women, could help others. So she wrote her book about how women can empower themselves in business. She has since written books on business and dating. She talks about how she went bankrupt and about her two years of only having her truck, her dog, and a cell phone after losing her business. She says she needed to get her story out there for her own satisfaction. "It was for me, and hopefully it will make a difference for someone else." Heather believes that many of us with ADHD have to put on a good face most of the time despite what's going on in our lives. And maybe that's a great quality, but she felt that her story could help others.

Heather is now coaching others on sales and online marketing. She's out speaking on the subject, and she feels that her life is heading in the right direction. She is also running a fitness supplement company with a partner called E2 Lab. She's confident and continues to create using her passion and her ADHD mind. Her coaching allows her to use her ADHD for good and growth. "I'm finally leveraging my ADD because I see and hear things that my clients don't see and hear.

"My strength is in creation and creating what's next. I really believe in my heart of hearts that entrepreneurs are creators and good entrepreneurs are ADD. I say go ADDers!"

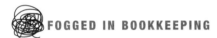 FOGGED IN BOOKKEEPING

If there is one part of my business that I actually hate, hands down it has to be the bookkeeping. I know "hate" is a strong word, but it's the truth. It's painful for me. And, quite honestly, my bookkeeping is not that complicated, since we bill for time. I like to say that I would rather be dragged over broken glass than do my bookkeeping.

And then there is Meghan Blair-Valero, who owns "Fogged in Bookkeeping," based in Nantucket, Massachusetts. You would think someone with ADHD owning a bookkeeping company would be a disaster, but Meghan found a business where her ADHD is actually an asset. She can see the big picture and then help that business with a larger snapshot of what's going on in the business. "I function in a high-level way," says Meghan. "I make a good C-level person because I can see the whole picture and run through the scenarios pretty far down the line. I think people with ADHD do that well." She feels that in some cases it's to their detriment, because it can bring on some anxiety, seeing too far down the road and then wondering how to handle certain situations.

But seeing what others do not see clearly has it advantages in business, she feels. "It works to your advantage in an entrepreneurial or C-level executive role because you're seeing further down the line. The things you worry about, other people don't even think about. The possibilities you see for something, other people don't see." It took her a while to realize that many around her needed some time to catch up to her thinking without getting frustrated.

Growing up, Meghan was a student who actually did very well, as opposed to others you have met who did not navigate school well. "I did academically really well, not because I was a driven student or a typical learner but because I was observant, figured out what game needed to be played to get the grade, and did it." In all of high school, even though she was an AP English student, she rarely read the books. She was a sight-reader, and that's how she got through school. She read books that she was assigned either in her own time frame or didn't read them at all. She would listen to the discussion of the book the next day in class. "If the point is to pass the test, that serves you well. However, in the long run in real life, it doesn't serve you real well."

What is ironic is that Meghan cofounded the Nantucket Book Festival, and now she is an avid reader. And she says that if you ask anyone about her, most people would say she is a big reader and that she loves books, without any knowledge of her past. "I've gone back as an adult and read the books that were assigned to me in high school that I didn't have the patience or wherewithal to read because I had a learning disability nobody knew and I couldn't read the pages as fast as they wanted me to read them in the time frame they wanted me to read them in. I would get frustrated and throw the book aside and say that I could pass the test." She graduated fourth in her class without actually doing much of the work.

She went on to college and was focusing her attention on arts education for children. During that time she was working for an arts program and was teaching a few days a week as she went to school. She picked up a few hours working in the office on the books as well. But the treasurer of the board of directors got to know her and gave her a little dose of reality. He said that being on Nantucket, there were maybe four art jobs open in the school system so that meant what she was going to school for didn't have a lot of job openings on a small island.

She went on to take a bookkeeping class to learn the software they were using, and she adapted to it very quickly. While she was still taking the course, she got her first client. Mind you, she hadn't even opened up the business yet. But a guy with the proverbial brown shopping bag of receipts came to her and asked her for her help with bookkeeping. She was also helping with the arts nonprofit, and she felt comfortable doing the organization's bookkeeping.

Still working for the nonprofit, Meghan and her boyfriend bought a house together, but soon after, he became ill and she found herself responsible for the mortgage and taking care of her young child. Her nonprofit salary was not going to cut it as a single wage earner. She started offering her bookkeeping services, and her business was officially launched. She left the job at the nonprofit, dropped out of school, and before she knew it, she had several paying clients. She says she never meant to start the business but did so out of necessity. In true ADHD fashion, she took a risk by dropping everything and starting a business without any guarantee of a paycheck. She needed the money to keep paying the bills, and she could have looked for a higher-paying job, but she decided to take the risk and go out on her own instead.

After a stressful couple of years growing the business, she finally took the opportunity to get an official diagnosis of ADHD. She says she was having trouble communicating with others, including the staff she hired, and it was frustrating. She was scattered and trying to lead a team as a fairly new business owner. She was late to appointments, which added to her frustration. "There are always three more things I can do before I walk out the door, or if I'm hyperfocused on something that I'm very interested in, time doesn't exist."

Like others with ADHD, Meghan needs to stay interested in what she is doing professionally. In the business, she started to look more at the overall health of these businesses and how they could do better. She took on a partner in a new venture called Eastern Light Advisors, which helps businesses with business development advice as well as guidance on seeking capital. It's a great venture for Meghan, as it allows her to be involved in many other businesses during the course of the year without the financial pressure of starting a business herself: "I get to start eight businesses a year." She feels fulfilled because she can be creative all the time and help another business grow with her ideas and insight. "I keep my ADHD brain happy because I'm doing something different all the time." She gets to apply the skill that comes with her ADHD brain of seeing how things are interconnected as well as seeing things that other people don't see.

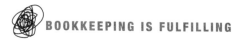 ## BOOKKEEPING IS FULFILLING

Meghan admits that there are not many out there who find bookkeeping their passion. What did happen, however, is that she woke up one day and realized that helping others and those in business was fulfilling. "I love taking the mess and making it tidy. Contrary to most people with ADHD, where they can live among the piles, I'm kind of the opposite. As an early coping skill, I found that if the bed is made and the room is picked up and there are fewer distractions, then I can focus on what I need to focus on. In business I feel that if the mess is cleaned up, then I can focus on what's important." And that's what she does for her clients: She and her staff clean up the mess of bookkeeping and help them move forward.

"I like helping other people succeed. I never once woke up and said I want to be a bookkeeper, but I did say that I knew I wanted to help people be successful. I found something I did well and enjoyed in that way. I didn't enjoy it for the numbers; I enjoyed it for how it made me feel."

But Meghan does have a bit of a different view on finding your way or your passion in life. "I think the idea of finding your passion and building something around it—that can be tough advice. I think if you can find something that you enjoy enough to do day in and day out, you can save your passion for photography or something else." Meghan feels that, in some cases, you can tire out your passion if you turn it into a business. I agree with her to some extent. There was a time when I could not dream of doing anything other than public relations. But then I found other ways to maintain passion for what I was doing.

"I think finding career paths that allow you the flexibility to be you without feeling the need to change yourself is huge. When I figured that out, I allowed myself to stop beating up on myself for not fitting the mold. And in my own way, not fitting the mold was benefiting me and it was benefiting others, so it was okay not to fit in the mold anymore and it actually became a positive." And that, Meghan says, is a huge builder of self-esteem.

CHAPTER TWELVE

lose the shame

I'm not going to end this book with a "suck it up"
or "just get over it" speech, because I know it's not that simple. But
just know that you think differently as a person with ADHD. With
ADHD come positives and negatives, and as Dr. Hallowell stated
earlier, we can only hope that the positives outweigh the negatives.
It's what we strive for. But please take one last dose of reality before
we part ways: You are not a moral failure. Your elementary school
report cards and comments of "not living up to his potential" do not
define you as an adult.

One thing people interviewed for this book have in common
is they have gotten out of their own way. And they didn't do it by
thinking poorly of themselves. We all have bad days, and we learn
how to make the best of them. So you sat on the sofa all day and
watched movies. Cut yourself some slack. Just get up and try to kick
ass the next day.

Michael B. says "dealing with ADD now is partly walking
through the fear of not being good enough." And he is correct, I
believe. Many of us keep those report cards and those visits to the
principal's office in our minds still, whether we know it or not, and
we have to tell ourselves that we are good enough and that we are,

in many cases, better equipped for some roles than others who may have gotten good grades in school. We doubt ourselves from time to time and wonder if there is an easier route. But you have to stay the course. You owe it to yourself.

For many with ADHD, however, it's not that simple, and there are things in your past that you'll need to work to overcome. Yes, you heard from your teachers to pay attention when you were gazing out the window, and you got in trouble when you brought home a bad report card. You may have even been the kid in school no one understood or were even bullied. But for many of us, our parents were overwhelmed. During the time when I grew up in the '70s, there was no official diagnosis for what we had. And when your parents don't have an accurate snapshot and some kind of diagnostic criteria to help them understand what you are going through, that can lead to stress and frustration. I believe this was evident in my house as a kid; many of the people I interviewed, who grew up in the same era, agree. ADHD kids are often frustrated, act out, and get into trouble. What happens after that? We were disciplined and yelled at. Over the years, we got yelled at more, and that can chip away at our self-esteem. When we got older, we suffered from shame. If this is still an issue for you, therapy can play a role. If you have things in your past that you need to sort out, you should consider that option.

Shame can be a big thing to overcome. Dr. David Nowell says that when new patients come into his office they conduct some preliminary grief work. "I think shame is the biggest obstacle in treating adults with ADHD because the very definition of ADHD involves a discrepancy between authority and performance." Dr. Nowell goes on to say that adults with ADHD have high energy and creativity as well as high aspirations. But performance can be spotty from day to day. For some, consistency is not there. We want to be successful, but we just have those days when those habits can get in the way of our full potential.

Dr. Timothy A. Pychyl says, "People who have chronic problems with attention or impulsivity can really beat themselves up all the time. We hear, 'I'm such a screwup' or 'I wish I wasn't like this.' And if you don't cut yourself some slack in terms of that self-compassion, you're never going to have the motivation to just try again. When you forgive yourself, you're more likely to try again."

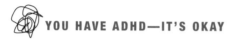 ## YOU HAVE ADHD—IT'S OKAY

Many adults with ADHD just dust themselves off and do it all over again the next day, as you have witnessed in this book. "With ADHD, we are the most resilient people I have ever known," says Dana Rayburn. "I can't imagine other people failing one day and then getting up the next and determining the day is going to be successful and doing that over and over again their whole lives, but that's what we do."

Dana says it's important to make sure you are looking at the positives of ADHD: "I think what makes someone successful is looking at the positives, building their world around their strengths and avoiding their weaknesses, instead of wallowing in those weaknesses. That's absolutely huge. So much of it is attitude, and so much of it is realizing that this is what I've been given and I've got to work with it and I've got to make my world work with it, instead of just wishing it were something else."

Dana says that she drops into some of these ADHD groups on Facebook sometimes, and as she puts it, it's heartbreaking. So many people are wallowing in the fact that they have ADHD and can't seem to get out of their own way. And I see a lot of it on other social networks, such as Twitter, where many focus on the negatives. We all have shitty days, whether we have ADHD or not. So many times, we just seem to let it affect us that much more. If you're one of these people, know that there are people like Dana and the many other professionals out there who can help guide you through your negatives and help you focus on the positives.

"Yeah, it's hard but it doesn't have to be that hard, and there are good things that come with it," Dana points out. "What good is it to just wallow in it as if this is the worst thing that ever happened to anybody? Yes, some people's lives are really screwed up because of their ADHD; I see it all the time. And what I also see with those people is that they don't tend to take responsibility and they don't really want to do what needs to be done to change."

Dana goes on to say that the people who are highly negative and don't want to put in the work necessary to change are the ones who are most resistant to change. They are the most resistant to finding a new path for themselves.

Wallowing in self-pitying because of your ADHD doesn't make it any better, but what does make your life with ADHD better is to figure out other ways around it. Dana recommends asking yourself, "What are my strengths, and what do I need to do to arrange my world so I can spend most of my time in my strengths?" She goes on to say that much of being successful with ADHD is a positive mind-set and a lot of self-awareness.

"I think once people step back and really learn about it and learn why they do what they do and understand it and understand the things they need to do to make their lives easier, then it's really kind of fun. I like being me. I like thinking the way that I do. Not every day—some days are tough—but 90 percent of the time, it's pretty darn fun to have my brain and my creativity. Life's interesting, and life's fun, and there's always something interesting going on, and I'm always learning something new. I'm always looking out that window."

Greg McDaniel says that for people to get comfortable they need to come to terms with their ADHD and do what's needed to be successful at life and at managing their symptoms. "First, they need to understand that they have ADHD and that it's okay." He says he feels that, for some, it may come as a shock, and their first tendency is to stick their head in the sand, but that's not the right approach. "You're not alone, there are tons of us out here, and it's actually not a bad thing." And Greg echoes what many others who have ADHD say—that it's not a disability. There are many abilities that come with being ADHD. "I have something that others do not, and that makes me special."

He also says that if you find you need medication, use it. Greg uses ADHD medication sparingly, but he says it does help. "I'm a big proponent of medication. It does help me, and I can feel a physical difference."

He notes that you should try medication, and don't try to tough it out yourself if you don't have to. For him, it does make a dramatic difference. "It allows me to home in and focus on the things I need to focus on, instead of being just all over the place."

Greg also says that it's very important for you to educate yourself about ADHD and what you can do to manage and thrive with it. Journaling helps as well. Take notes on the things that you struggle with, write down the positives and negatives, and then you have the information you need to try to make the necessary changes in your life. He says he has practiced this, and it has been very helpful in his life.

Greg says that you need to face the fact that you have ADHD and that life is going to go on and you'll need to make the most out of what you have been given. Sure, you had a less than desirable time in school and, like Greg, maybe you flipped over a few desks in elementary school, but don't let that define you. "It doesn't make you inferior to anyone else; it doesn't make them better than you; and it doesn't give them more abilities to succeed in life or in work or relationships. The thing that's not going to work is you not understanding how to live with ADHD."

Learning anything can be a challenge with ADHD, and it can set off a ton of frustration, which leads to anger and shame in many cases. Greg, who has ADHD and dyslexia, has always had challenges learning, but he has found ways of getting the knowledge he wants and needs, and he says that with those two issues, reading was not a fulfilling experience growing up. "Find the way you want to learn and then learn that way." Many of us, especially in school, just needed to be taught in a way that our brains would absorb. For myself, I find that to be true even today.

Greg feels that you don't have to learn in a traditional manner to be successful, and I completely agree. I would have to say that pretty much everything I have learned about conducting PR and video marketing campaigns for my business has been self-taught. I didn't go to school for public relations, and I have never taken a course on video production.

Heather Ann Havenwood says that those with ADHD need to dream big and state out loud what they want to the world. But she also says that, in some cases, know that when you do, you may get all the naysayers telling you that you can't reach that big dream or goal. She calls this one of the journeys of ADHD: knowing that when you do state a huge goal or dream, in many cases, others around you might not see what you see. Guess what? That's okay. In fact, maybe that's a good thing!

Heather has a quote that she refers to daily when she starts a project or an important endeavor. She asks herself this: "Does this feed my confusion or strengthen my clarity?" She says, "There was definitely a time in my life where I was just swirling and I didn't know which way to go. And things are coming at you and sometimes when you are swirling, you're just grabbing versus being grounded." She feels that it's an emotional conversation with yourself, and if you ask that question, your energy and body will give you the answer. "For someone with ADD, who loves the shiny object, that's definitely saved me.

Because when you are coming from a place of clarity in anything your life, you're coming from a place of strength. And when you're coming from a place of strength, you just have the ability to become more successful."

Heather also believes that many with ADHD do have issues with self-worth. Once again, we were told growing up to try harder and focus and all the other things grown-ups said to us when they felt we were not living up to our potential. As we have mentioned countless times, that has stuck with us, even as adults. I believe that, as adults, we doubt ourselves in some situations and we have to trust our judgment and our own self-worth. Heather has one more quote that is very important to her: "Never stay where your presence is not valued." She equates it to being at a party or an event where you might not feel as if you are being acknowledged at all. "Don't prove yourself, just remove yourself." Heather admits that while it might not be so much of an ADHD trait, this statement and practice have grounded her and taught her a lot about herself.

I really do agree with her philosophy because it's very stressful to try to fit in and to constantly prove yourself to someone else. I can somewhat relate this to my own business. I carefully choose the clients I work with and make sure that I can provide what they're looking for. While most clients value your background and expertise, some question everything and even tell you how to do your job. As Heather says, it's important to feel as if you and the service you're providing are valued, and that also helps you stay focused.

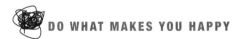 **DO WHAT MAKES YOU HAPPY**

I'm confident in saying that if you are doing what you love and it makes you happy, that goes a long way in creating a fulfilling life. Dan Nainan is a very successful comedian, who just happens to have ADHD. Dan's story is one of persistence and discovering what he was really good at. Dan was an engineer at Intel. He was responsible for designing and creating technical presentations for the company. The only problem was he had a fear of speaking in public. He was very confident in the technical aspects of the presentation, but when the audience numbered in the thousands, he got a little nervous.

To get over that fear, he took a comedy class. The final test for the class was to perform at a popular comedy club in San Francisco. After his coworkers saw the tape of his performance, he was asked to do some comedy at the annual sales conference and had the entire room laughing. He went on to perform at the company's annual meeting in front of over two thousand employees and was a big hit there as well.

Dan took a risk and went out to find his way in the comedy world: a guy who at one time was scared of speaking in public. He now travels all over the world, performed on NBC's *Last Comic Standing*, and has done comedy routines for President Barack Obama and countless other Washington politicians over the past several years.

During his time at Intel, he was working with another presenter who was doing stand-up comedy. Before he took that class, his friend suggested that whenever he came across a good story or something funny, he should write it down. Dan took his advice and when he got to the comedy class, he had a stack of jokes on cards. At first he got a lot of laughs when he told his jokes in the class, but the second time around, no one laughed. He says he came very close to quitting the class. "I don't know what it is that made me keep going," says Dan. "Maybe because I had quit so many things in my life and never finished anything. I don't know what drove me to stay in that class, but doing so changed my life."

Dan clearly found a career that he loves. Who wouldn't love going around the country, telling jokes, and having people laugh?

One thing people with ADHD crave is that praise from others, so a career in comedy could be great career for those with ADHD. And while Dan says he did enjoy working for Intel, he didn't think twice before making the jump to build his next career and hasn't regretted it.

Dan suggests that if you are trying to find that next thing in your life, try to do it on the side. Many of us quit our jobs and just go for it, myself included, but if you can't quite make the leap yet, explore your options during your free time. He recommends giving up the countless hours of watching television and going to parties, or whatever it is you've been doing with your leisure time, and devote it instead to finding what's next in your life. "In any major city in America and also because of the Internet, you can take classes in anything your heart desires."

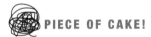 **PIECE OF CAKE!**

Monique Akeman runs a specialty cake business in Massachusetts. I have had her cakes and other products, and I can honestly say they are some of the best I have ever tasted. If you ask me, she found her calling. Monique says that, growing up, she was pretty good in school, but admits it was harder than it may have appeared. A lack of cognitive processing caused her to stay in for hours doing her homework while other kids in the neighborhood were out playing, having already completed theirs. She says some days it took her three to six hours to do a simple assignment. "Academically I did well, but the side that no one really understood was how much more effort I put into it just to get a normal result."

Socially, Monique says she was a "hot mess." She says she always kind of spoke her mind, which in the beginning kids were attracted to. But she noticed that her friends would suddenly desert her after playing with her enthusiastically for a while, and she wondered what she had done to make them go away. She feels that when she was a child, she was not really aware of certain social cues. She also points out that because she is Hispanic, she was not treated like other kids growing up, which led to even more social stress. She feels that other kids in her Girl Scout troop, for example, only tolerated her. She says it was bad enough that she had ADHD growing up, but then the color of her skin only complicated things.

Monique got the itch to bake cakes after seeing cakes being decorated at a large grocery warehouse store. There was a woman behind the glass decorating the cakes, and she says she would spend hours watching her create them. "I was mesmerized," says Monique. "I'll never forget it. It was so amazing to see something go from nothing to something beautiful." She began to makes cakes on her own for various occasions and continued to teach herself the craft. "To this day, I can't dress myself to save my life or put an outfit together." But she says that she finds decorating cakes so simple.

When her daughter was old enough to go to preschool, she started taking a course on cakes, and as she puts it, the rest is history—and her cake business was born. She loves the design part, and if you ever get a chance to see her cakes, you can see just how creative she is. "Somebody comes to me with an idea, and I get to dream it up. I get to take whatever their theme is and just go crazy with it." She says that she takes that idea, then translates it to make the cake practical, functional, and cost-effective. "I think I always was creative but was so busy trying to keep up with the academics and trying to fit in that it wasn't harnessed." As far as creating incredible cakes and using her ADHD, Monique says, "I don't see it so much as feeding my brain as letting my brain go. When I'm decorating or designing, it's just about letting my brain go, and it's almost like I can breathe." She says she doesn't have to worry about all the other things looming in her head about the business.

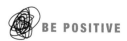 **BE POSITIVE**

If you're new to ADHD, you will probably, if you haven't already, go on the Internet and do some searching. You'll most likely stumble on the CDC website, where the first line says that ADHD is a serious public health issue. It goes on to crush the idea that people with ADHD have contributed much to our society, the world of business, our economy, and more. Yes, growing up with ADHD can suck at times, but if we continue to say it's a crisis rather than taking the time to uncover the positive aspects of this condition, if that's what you want to call it, then we will continue to quash the creativity and contributions of future adults with ADHD. What the CDC also says is that the number of diagnoses of ADHD continues to grow in the United States. That means that more kids will enter adulthood with ADHD.

Your job as an adult with ADHD is to find every way possible to manage your ADHD, survive with it, and thrive with it. I know it's easy to get down on yourself and tell yourself you're not good enough. We have all been there. But you have just met a group of people who are not only managing their ADHD, but thriving with it. They are using it to bring new products and services to market; and they are helping others to dispel the notion that this is only a public health issue, because it's not. Harnessed and developed properly, you can do amazing things with your ADHD.

If you are still procrastinating on kicking a little ass with your type of brain, Dr. Timothy Pychyl said one thing to me before we ended our phone interview for this book: "The only limited resource that you and I truly have is time on this planet. And we don't know how much we're going to get, so to waste any of it is deeply sinful and at least deeply problematic. It's so desperately important to live our lives while we can. It's not a dress rehearsal." Don't procrastinate on the next phase of your life!

Here you'll find many valuable resources to help
you with your ADHD, including websites, apps, blogs and podcasts, and contact information for many in this book.

ORGANIZATIONS

CHADD: *Children and Adults with Attention Deficit Hyperactivity Disorder.* http://www.chadd.org/ and http://help4adhd.org/

Meetup: *Find an ADHD meeting or support group in your area.*
http://www.meetup.com/

ADDitude: Magazine offering strategies and support for ADHD.
http://www.additudemag.com/

ADDA: *Attention Deficit Disorder Association.*
http://add.org/

NIMH: *National Institute of Mental Health.*
http://www.nimh.nih.gov

ADHD COACHES AND DOCTORS

Dr. Edward Hallowell: http://www.drhallowell.com/

Dana Rayburn: http://danarayburn.com/

Jay Carter: http://www.hyperfocusedcoaching.com

Jonathan Carroll: http://adhdefcoach.com/

Eric Tivers: http://www.erictivers.com/

Brendan Mahan: http://www.adhdessentials.com

David Nowell: http://www.drnowell.com/

Melissa Orlov: https://www.adhdmarriage.com/

BUSINESS AND ENTREPRENEURIAL COACHES

Chris Berlow: https://www.empoweredmastery.com/
Heather Havenwood: http://heatherhavenwood.com/

PODCASTS AND BLOGS

Faster Than Normal with Peter Shankman: http://fasterthannormal.
com
ADHD reWired with Eric Tivers: www.ADHDrewired.com
Distraction with Dr. Edward Hallowell: http://www.distractionpod-
cast.com/
ADHD and Marriage with Melissa Orlov & Dr. Edward Hallowell:
https://www.adhdmarriage.com/
iProcrastinate with Dr. Timothy Pychyl: http://iprocrastinate.libsyn.
com/
The ADHD Nerd by Ryan McRae: http://www.theadhdnerd.com

APPS

Evernote: https://evernote.com
Pomodoro Technique: http://pomodorotechnique.com/
WeDo: WeDo.com
Wunderlist: https://www.wunderlist.com/

ACKNOWLEDGMENTS

I would like to acknowledge all the people with ADHD who took part in this book. For many of us growing up, we never spoke about the fact that we had ADHD. Some of us hid the fact and many of us even doubted whether there was something a bit different about us. I believe it is a huge step for some of us to tell our stories and show a somewhat vulnerable side of ourselves. Many in this book reached out to me and told me they wanted to tell their story and hopefully help others with ADHD.

Of course, I need to acknowledge my wife Emily as she has put up with my career changes every ten years as well as the countless unfinished projects around the house. Hey, I'm not perfect . . .

There have been several people in my life who have allowed me to learn and grow without a college degree. The first, of course, would be my father and my mother, who passed away at the age of sixty-nine. I believe my father followed a traditional path, working in pretty much the same career field for much of his life. Me? Well, you read my story.

My mother for many years was a stay-at-home mom and I challenged her every day as a child. There were days when hyperactivity was probably an understatement to describe my energy, and I'm quite confident I exhausted her patience on those days.

But as I grew older my parents let me chart my own course and fail at times, and because of that, I learned more than I could have ever absorbed in a classroom or lecture hall. We all learn differently, and they recognized that.

In my professional life I must acknowledge Bob Johnson, former CEO of Special Olympics Massachusetts. Bob was well aware that I did not possess a college degree, but he believed in my passion and abilities. After revamping the public relations program of the organization, he gave me a shot at becoming a vice president in charge of fundraising and marketing when the job description clearly stated a college degree was required.

And as they say, last but certainly not least, is Master Chris Berlow, whom you met in this book. Chris worked with me over the years as a business and life coach and a friend. He was a major influence as I wrote this book. Chris pushed me at just the right tone and speed in order for me to accomplish many things, including this book and what lies ahead in my life.

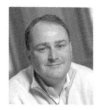

David Greenwood lives just outside of Boston, Massachusetts, with his wife and son. On the drug Ritalin for many of his childhood years, David was hyperactive, unfocused, and faced many academic challenges in school, including flunking out freshman year at a vocational high school—a clear case of ADHD.

An entrepreneur at heart, he owns Street Smart PR/Video, a small public relations and video marketing firm. Over the years, David has owned other small businesses including a karate school, as well as a popular restaurant in suburban Boston. With the exception of twelve years, he has always been self-employed as an adult.

As a person with ADHD, he feels ADHD has always fueled his desire to be his own boss. For him, ADHD has given him a creative and energetic edge in the business world. In writing *Overcoming Distractions*, he set out to find others who also felt that ADHD was, in fact, a gift if managed properly.

David has always been driven to create his own path to success, and he wanted to tell the stories of other successful people with ADHD.